Hand And Forearm Exercises

Grip Strength Workout And Training Routine

Patrick Barrett

BarrettBooks.com

Copyright © 2012 Patrick Barrett

All rights reserved.

ISBN-10: 1479143782
ISBN-13: 978-1479143788

CONTENTS

Introduction	1
What Can Hand And Forearm Exercise Do For You?	4
Warming Up And Stretching	7
The Exercises	9
Grippers	11
Isometrics	18
Block Weights	29
Walking Broom	42
Sledgehammer	45
Hanging	52
Farmer's Carry	54
Gyro Ball	56
Handstands	65
Dumbbell Twist	70
Fingertip Pushups And Planks	72
Rope Climbing	76
Rolling Towels	81

Schedule And Recovery	85
Connect With Me	88
Conclusion	90
Books By Patrick Barrett	92
About The Author	93

> "If you have a fine, warm, strong handclasp, it will create a favorable impression with those whom you meet... A good grip is a fine thing to possess."

-Bob Hoffman, Strength & Health Magazine, August 1943

Books by Patrick Barrett:

Natural Exercise: Basic Bodyweight Training and Calisthenics for Strength and Weight-Loss

Advanced Bodyweight Exercises: An Intense Full Body Workout In A Home Or Gym

The Natural Diet: Simple Nutritional Advice For Optimal Health In The Modern World

How To Do A Handstand: From the Basic Exercises To The Free Standing Handstand Pushup

Easy Exercises: Simple Workout Routine For Busy People In The Office, At Home, Or On The Road

Best Ab Exercises: Abdominal Workout Routine For Core Strength And A Flat Stomach

One Arm Pull Up: Bodyweight Training And Exercise Program For One Arm Pull Ups And Chin Ups

Hand And Forearm Exercises: Grip Strength Workout And Training Routine

Disclaimer:

This book was not written or reviewed by a doctor, personal trainer, dietitian, or other licensed person. Always consult with your doctor before beginning any exercise routine or implementing any change in your diet or medication.

INTRODUCTION

Hi! I'm Patrick Barrett, and I'd like to thank you for purchasing this book.

I'm glad that you've decided to dedicate some time to hand, grip strength, and forearm exercise. These often-overlooked exercises can be very rewarding, and their effects can be far-reaching—in fact, if you can successfully strengthen your hands, you can probably harness more of the upper-body strength you've already got that might be going to waste. More on that in the next chapter.

I first became interested in hand strength as a wrestler in high school. My technique wasn't exactly perfect, but I found that just by maintaining a firm grip on my opponent's wrists, arms, or waist, I could considerably limit his movements and create an advantage for myself.

Even if you aren't a wrestler, this basic idea applies to many athletic situations, since almost every sport depends on your ability to use your hands—whether you're holding a baseball bat, a football, a basketball, a hockey stick, a tennis racket, a lacrosse stick, or a number of other pieces of equipment, your hands are what you use to control and direct the objects you use to play your game.

Stronger hands means better control and better performance—it's that simple. And when other players overlook this type of training, you have an opportunity to create an advantage for yourself.

But the benefits of hand and forearm training are not limited to athletes. Working on grip strength might be the single type of training that translates best to everyday life. When it comes to opening jars, carrying groceries, chopping vegetables, moving furniture, doing yardwork, even typing, having strong and healthy hands means you get things done quicker and better.

Face it—in everyday life, you seldom have to bench press or squat something. The muscles in your hands and forearms might be the ones you use most often, in sports and in life, and investing some time in keeping them strong and healthy will pay off, both in the short term, and years down the road.

In this book, we'll talk about exactly what stronger hands can do for you. Then we'll talk about what you should do before hand training to make sure your hands are limber and ready to work. We'll talk about a number of different exercises, many of which can be done with items around the house or with no equipment at all.

After that, we'll discuss how to incorporate hand and forearm exercise into your regular routine, and how to handle common issues you might run into.

Thanks again for purchasing this book. I'm confident that your grip strength training will be some of the most worthwhile and rewarding exercise that you do.

Other Books by Patrick Barrett:

Natural Exercise: Basic Bodyweight Training and Calisthenics for Strength and Weight-Loss

Advanced Bodyweight Exercises: An Intense Full Body Workout In A Home Or Gym

The Natural Diet: Simple Nutritional Advice For Optimal Health In The Modern World

How To Do A Handstand: From the Basic Exercises To The Free Standing Handstand Pushup

Best Ab Exercises: Abdominal Workout Routine For Core Strength And A Flat Stomach

Easy Exercises: Simple Workout Routine For Busy People In The Office, At Home, Or On The Road

One Arm Pull Up: Bodyweight Training And Exercise Program For One Arm Pull Ups And Chin Ups

WHAT CAN HAND AND FOREARM EXERCISE DO FOR YOU?

Your hands are critical in so many different physical activities because they are often the actual point of contact between your body and whatever you're picking up, throwing, hitting, or otherwise interacting with. Your hands are what actually "delivers" your strength, and if they aren't strong enough, then some measure of your effort is being wasted.

To illustrate the point, imagine that you have a truck that's towing a one thousand pound load. Imagine that the truck is strong enough to pull a five thousand pound load. This one thousand pound load should be no problem, right?

Now imagine that the only way you can attach the load to the truck is by using a chain that can only handle a one hundred pound load. See what I'm getting at here? Once you get above a hundred pounds, all that extra strength in the truck is irrelevant. You could put tons of new equipment into the truck to make it more and more powerful, but it won't make a bit of difference in the actual work it can do until you get a stronger chain.

The same goes for your body—you could have all the strength in the world in your back, chest, and shoulders, but if you're counting on weak hands to deliver it, you're out of luck.

Let's assume that you're a baseball player, and you want to hit the ball harder. So you develop your chest, arms, and shoulders so that you can have more power when you swing the bat.

Well, if your hands aren't strong enough to hold on to the bat when you connect with the ball, all that power you built up in your upper body is useless because your hands can't hold on enough to deliver that power to the ball. Even if you don't drop the bat, just being unable to maintain a firm grip when you connect means that the bat will 'give' a lot, and much of the power you're trying to deliver will never actually reach its target.

Or what if you're a linebacker? Let's imagine that you spend plenty of time on full-body exercise so that you can have the strength you need to fight past your opponents and reach the ball carrier. If your hands aren't strong enough to push away blockers, or to hold on to whomever you're trying to tackle, then all your strength is almost meaningless.

As you might guess, we could go on and on with this sort of scenario, but I think you see what I'm talking about here. In reality, it's not likely that your hands are so weak that all your other strength is worthless, but it is very likely —especially if you don't spend any time training your hands and forearms specifically—that your hand strength is lagging behind the rest of your body.

If your hands are not as strong as the rest of you, that means your body can't perform up to its potential.

It also means that you could see bigger gains in overall strength right in the beginning, because in addition to your hands themselves getting stronger, you'll finally be fully realizing the strength you already had, but weren't completely able to use.

Again, this doesn't just apply in sports. Strong, healthy hands are a great physical asset to have in ordinary daily life, not to mention in later years. Keeping your hands in good shape means less likelihood that you'll deal with the joint pain and other issues that many people experience as they get older.

So what does this all mean? Just that the time you spend developing strong hands is one of the best investments you can make in your body, regardless of your situation. With that in mind, let's get down to business—first we'll talk about warming up and stretching your hands, and then we'll take a look at the exercises.

WARMING UP AND STRETCHING

It's important in any workout routine to warm up and stretch your muscles, and your hands and forearms and no exception. We'll look at a couple quick things you should do before a hand workout to make sure you get the best results and minimize risk of injury.

Since you always want to warm up before you stretch—don't stretch cold muscles—we'll look at that first. The odds are good that your hands are semi-warm already, since you just tend to use your hands over the course of the day. To get them a little more ready for your workout, simply open your hands up and spread your fingers out all the way, then close them into fists. Repeat this ten times or so.

Then, lightly shake your hands out for a few seconds. That just helps loosen up your hands a bit more, and further stimulates blood flow.

Next, do these stretches:

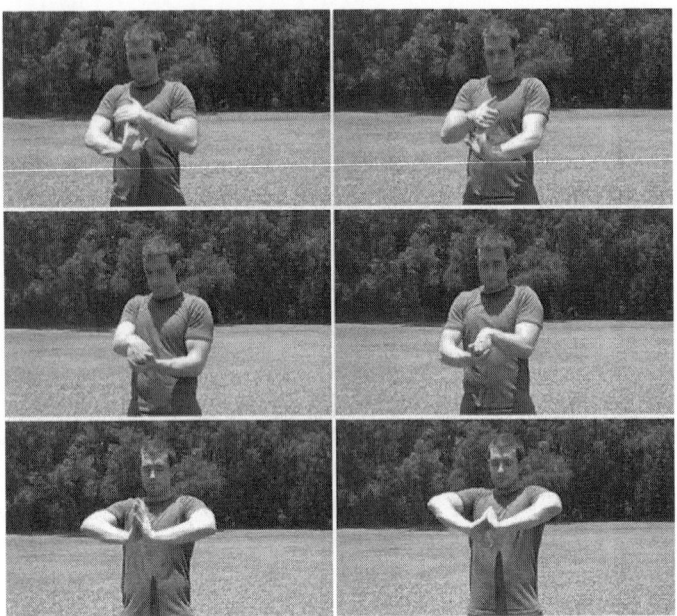

Apply light pressure so you can feel the stretch in your fingers as well as your forearms, and hold each position for ten seconds or so. Be sure to do all your warm ups and stretches equally on both hands.

That's it! Your hands should be warm and stretched and ready to go. If you plan on doing anything really heavy in your workout, you should do some light sets of that exercise for further warm up, but other than that you're ready for action. Let's look at the exercises.

THE EXERCISES

We're going to cover a lot of different types of exercises here. There are some that require no equipment at all; these are a great option because you can do them almost anywhere at almost any time.

Others require an ordinary household object, like a broom or a towel; you should have no problem doing these in most situations.

A few require relatively inexpensive pieces of equipment, ranging from a few dollars to twenty or thirty dollars.

My recommendation is that you try every single one of these exercises at least a couple of times, because every one has value and every one can make you stronger.

If you take advantage of all the exercises in this book, you can develop very, very strong hands. Just follow the directions carefully, make sure that you are using the right form, and then once you are used to the exercises, be sure to increase the difficulty from there.

We'll start with a look at grippers.

GRIPPERS

Hand grippers are sort of the classic hand strength training tool, and almost everyone has heard of them, including people who aren't even very much into hand training, or exercise in general.

You can probably go into your local Target or Wal-Mart and buy a pair of hand grippers for a few dollars. Let me tell you right now that you don't want to waste your time with those; they are far too easy to close to be effective.

The only worthwhile grippers that I know of are the Captains of Crush grippers made and sold by Iron Mind, which you can get from their website, or from Amazon.com or a few other places; with shipping charges from some sites (some cost more but have free shipping) one gripper usually ends up being a little less than 30 bucks.

At the time that I write this there are 11 different grippers for sale, each at a different level of difficulty, from 60

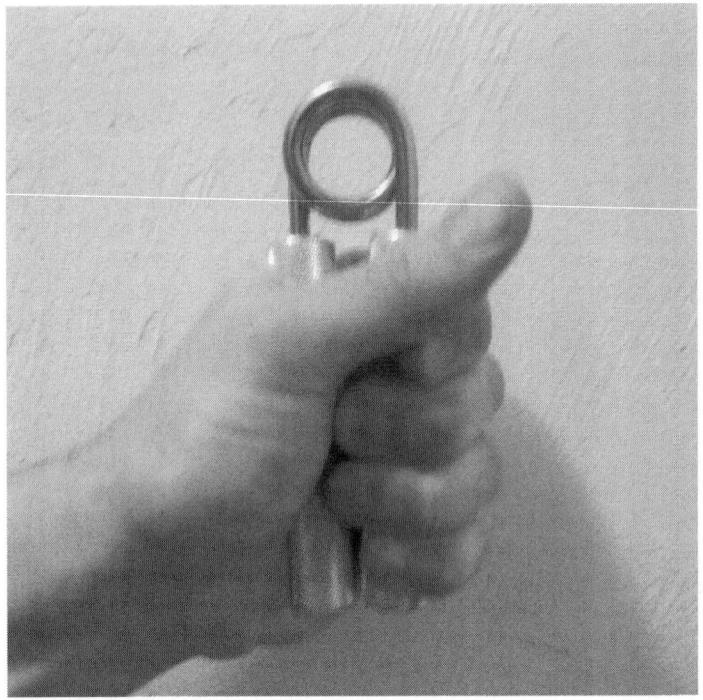

pounds all the way up to 365 pounds of pressure required to close them. There are four main grippers (conveniently named the 1, 2, 3, and 4). Closing the 3 and 4 grippers is so difficult that if you can do it, Iron Mind will send somebody out to certify you, and they will put your name on their official list.

Only five people have ever officially closed the number 4 (as I write this), and the last one was eight years ago, just to give you an idea of the level of difficulty. Also, they recently began certifying women who could close the number 2, and so far one woman has been able to.

So that's a little background info on these grippers, now we'll talk about actually using them.

First of all, here's a picture showing how to hold and close the gripper. Note that 'closing' means actually causing the two handles to touch. "Almost there" is good, but it doesn't count.

Some people really get into training with grippers, and some people prefer other methods. If this sounds at all interesting to you, you should probably pick up the Sport or Trainer gripper (two of the lower-end grippers) and get in some work with them.

If you like them, you can invest in some of the more challenging ones and try to work your way up the line. If you're not as into them, you can continue to use the grippers you have to mix up your workout a little bit while focusing on other exercises. Here's a few sample workouts you can do with these grippers:

Difficult Gripper

If you've got a gripper you can almost close, or you can only close it once or twice, this is a good approach.

First, be sure you're thoroughly warmed up, either on a lower-level gripper or with other exercise. If you can barely close this gripper, or you can only close it a couple of times, you're obviously exerting yourself a lot and you need to be well warmed up to perform well and avoid injury.

A basic, decent approach is to attempt one to three sets of 2-5 repetitions, with a couple of minutes of rest in between.

I know we just said this is a gripper you can close, at most, a couple of times, so when I say 2-5 repetitions, I really mean 2-5 attempts. If you can't close it even once, stick with 2 or 3 attempts to close it as much as possible. If you can close it one or two times, add another one to three attempts in there to round out the exercise.

When you fail to close, you can either do a partial repetition or an assisted repetition. A partial repetition means simple trying to close the gripper, failing, and releasing your hold. Obviously, your goal over time is for these partial reps to come closer and closer to successful attempts.

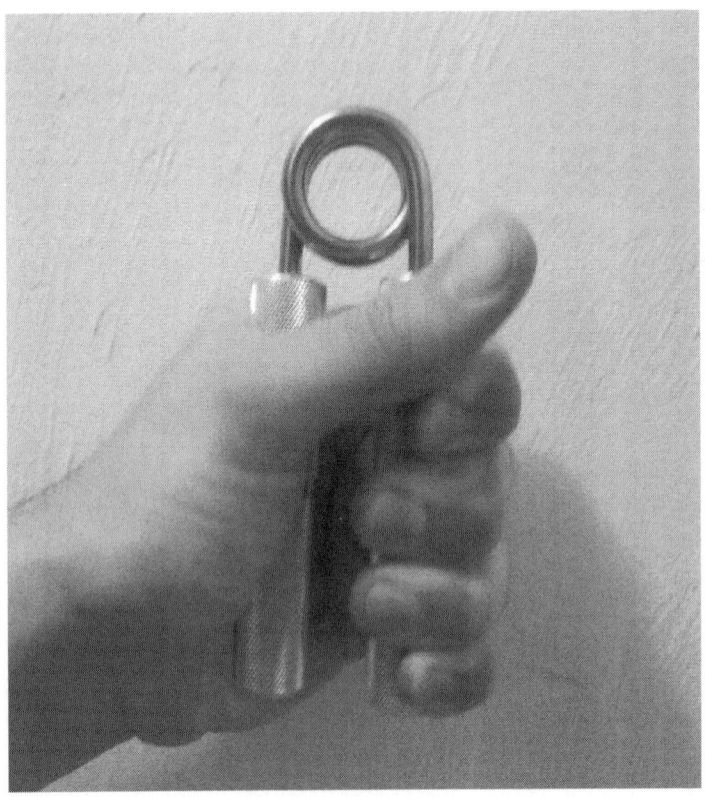

The other option is an assisted repetition. In this method, you close the gripper as much as possible with one hand, and then you bring in the other hand to assist in completing the close. If you can't close the gripper even with two hands, you should probably be working on a lower level gripper that is less challenging.

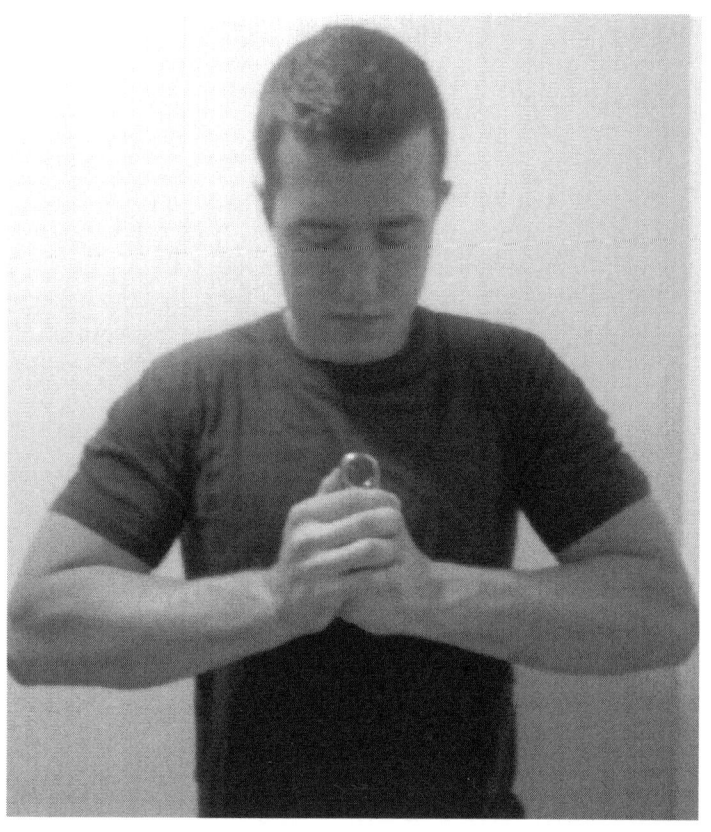

As you can see, you will put the palm of the assisting hand opposite the palm of the gripping hand. Then, using the muscles in your arms and chest, push your palms toward each other, while continuing to squeeze with the gripping hand, to close the gripper.

To get the most out of your assisted reps, try to do as much of the closing as possible with the gripping hand, and only use your assisting hand as much as you have to in order to close the gripper.

If you prefer one method over the other (partial reps versus assisted reps), feel free to use that method for the most part, but for best results you should mix in both at one time or another. On the one hand assisted reps allow for a complete range of motion, and they allow your gripping hand to max out through the end of the rep, but on the other hand, partial reps allow you to do as much work as possible with only the gripping hand, and they let you know how close you are to your goal.

Try them both out and see what you prefer, but plan to use both to some degree.

Moderate Gripper

Try this if you can close the gripper for 5-10 repetitions.

Do 3-6 sets of 5-10 repetitions with a couple of minutes of rest in between (for more reps, do fewer sets; for fewer reps, do more sets). For added difficulty, you can finish each set by holding the gripper closed for a few seconds. By the end you should have trouble closing the gripper for as many reps as you did in your first set; just round out the set with partial or assisted repetitions.

If you can do the full number of repetitions for each set, you should increase the repetitions, or the number of sets, or move to a harder gripper.

Easy Gripper

If you can get 10 full repetitions or more on a gripper, then you probably need something more challenging. Still, this can be a good gripper for a warm up, light exercise, or to supplement a larger routine incorporating other exercises.

For a warm up, light exercise, or as part of a larger routine, do 1-3 sets of 10-20 reps.

For an added challenge on this gripper (or any other gripper you can close fully), try to hold the gripper closed for as long as you can. This can be a great twist to add to your routine.

To increase the difficulty, insert a thin object between the handles (like a credit card or penny) and try to hold it there for as long as you can. You can also insert something with a little more grip to it (like a leather strap or a rope), and either attach weights to the strap or rope, or just try to pull it out with your other hand while still using your primary hand to hold the gripper closed around it.

******

So, now you've got a feel for these grippers, and you know some basic routines you can use. Some people get very serious with these grippers, and if you choose to do that you'll be able to find a huge number of different workouts and variations to work on.

If you're mildly to moderately interested, though, this should be enough information to keep you busy and to get your hands much stronger.

ISOMETRICS

There are a lot of ways that you can use isometrics to exercise your hands. The following is a simple routine that I came up with a few years ago which allows you to get a pretty complete hand and forearm workout anywhere, at any time.

It consists of eight different positions which you hold for ten seconds each, and you can do it through once, or a few times in a row, or a few times throughout the day, or just whenever you think of it. I like to do it when I'm standing in line, taking a walk, watching TV, and so on.

Before we describe this series, let's do one thing real quick: hold your arm straight out to your side.

Not too exciting, right?

Okay, now hold your arm straight out to your side again. This time, tense every muscle in your arm, from you shoulder out to your fingertips. Do you feel all that tension, and all those muscles working? Even though your arm is in the same position it was in before, now all the muscles are working hard.

That's the kind of tension you're going to need in your forearm, hand, and particularly your fingers when you do these isometric exercises. If you don't concentrate on flexing all the associated muscles, you won't get much out of this.

Learning to flex ALL the muscles involved, and to keep them flexed for the full allotted time, is a skill in itself—and as you keep doing these exercises you'll get better and better at it, and you'll get more out of the exercises.

Keep that in mind. Let's take a look.

Position 1

Hold your hand in the position pictured. Maintain tension in your thumb as well as your index and pinky finger, while squeezing your middle finger and ring finger together as hard you can.

Why do this? Well, if you're having trouble believing this will be beneficial, just take your other hand and grab your forearm around the meatiest part, a little closer to your elbow than to your wrist. Lay your fingers on top of you forearm, curl your thumb around to the underside of your forearm, and squeeze it slightly.

Now, squeeze your middle finger and ring finger together on your exercising hand, as just described.

Do you feel those muscles tensing up deep in your forearm? You can do the same thing with the other hand

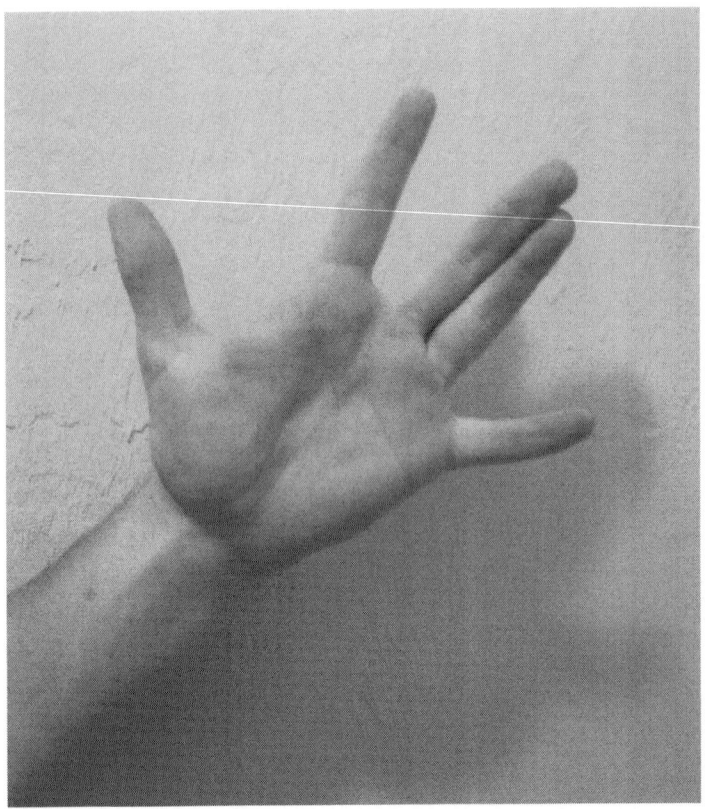

positions in this series; grab your forearm with your other hand, and you can feel the muscles working in your forearm when you do these isometrics.

You may need to slide your hand up and down your forearm a bit to feel which muscles are working, because different positions will focus on different parts of your forearm, but rest assured that these simple isometric exercises are giving you a good workout—and if you're still skeptical, just give it a shot anyway, and you'll feel it once you're done.

You may just feel like you're squeezing your fingers together in different ways, but lots of muscular activity is taking place throughout your entire forearm.

Position 2

Immediately after the previous position, hold your hands in the position pictured. Maintain tension in your thumb, and press your pinky and ring finger together while simultaneously pressing your index and middle fingers together.

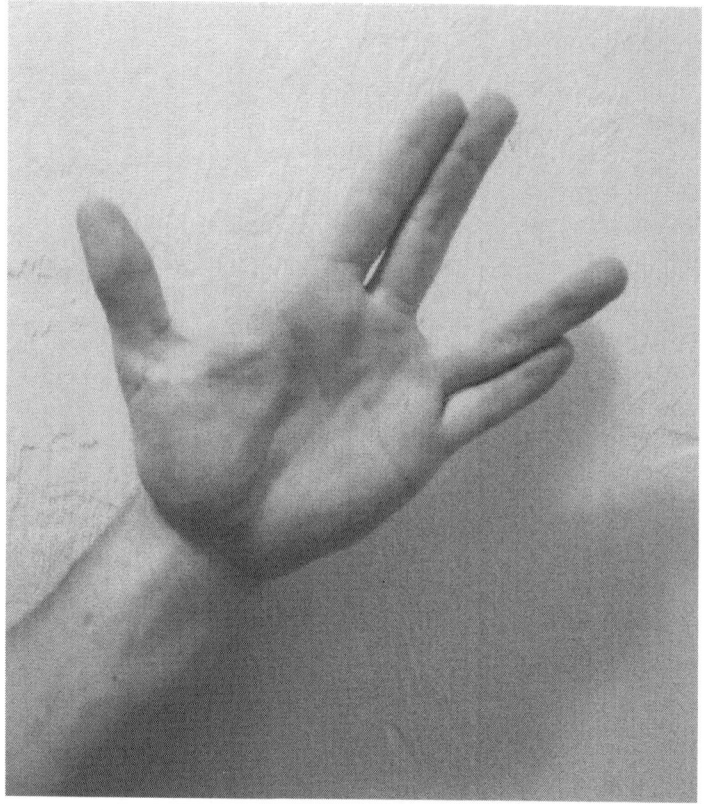

Position 3

Now bring all your fingers and your thumb together, and press them all together against each other.

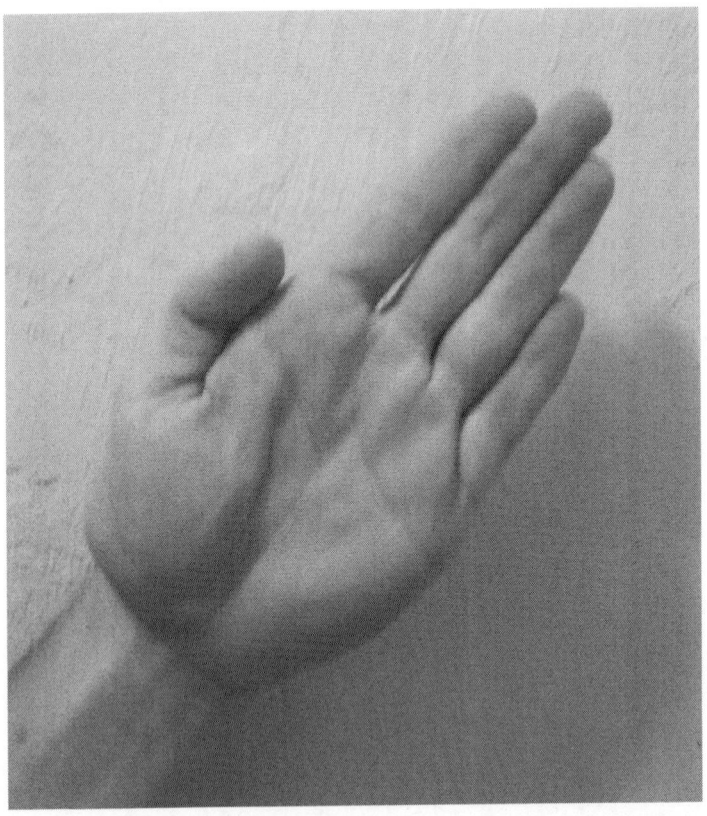

Position 4

Next, spread all your fingers outward and maintain tensions throughout your hand and fingers.

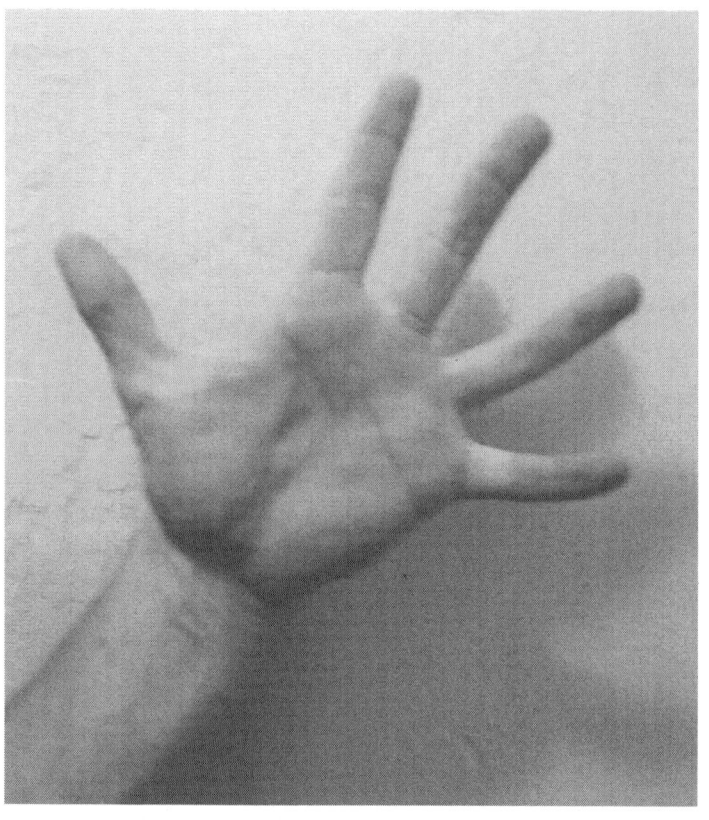

Position 5

Now, squeeze your hand hard in a fist. Be sure to squeeze each individual finger, as well as your thumb, and keep up the tension in your whole hand.

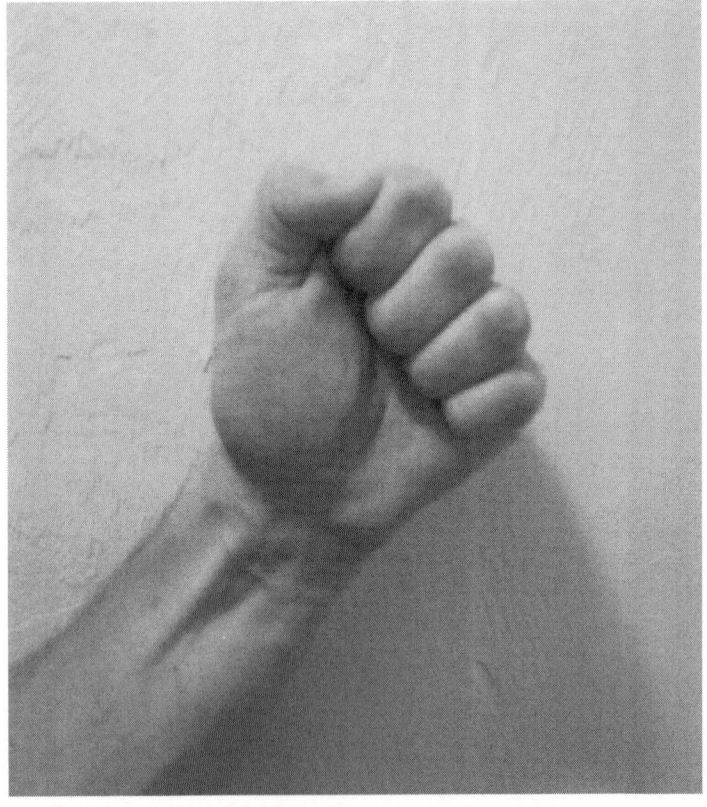

Position 6

Next, open your hand out wide; this time don't just spread your fingers out, but back as well, as though you're trying to open your hand as wide as possible.

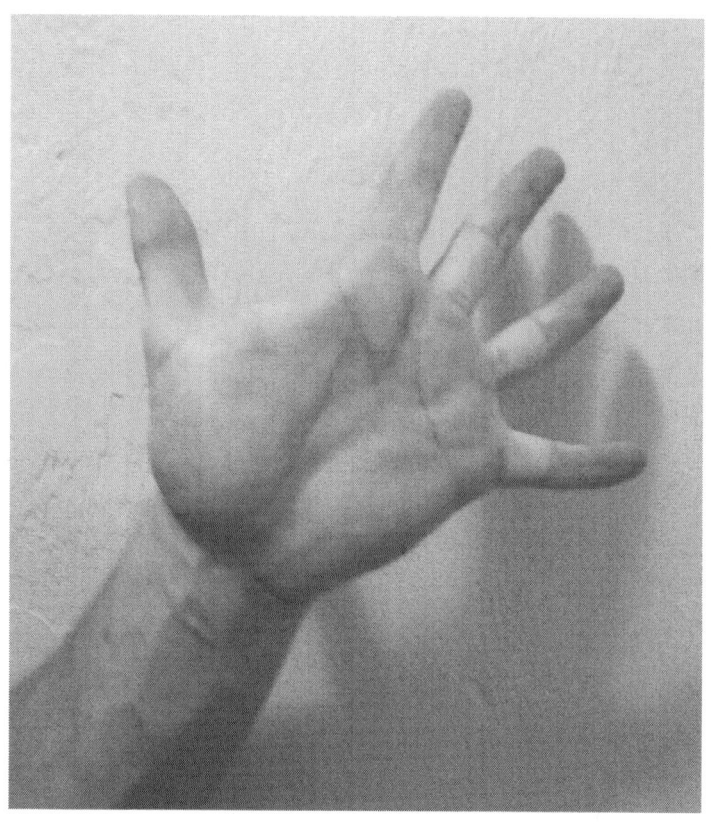

Position 7

For this position, curl your wrist as far forward as you can, and then in that position do your best to squeeze your fist like you did in position 5.

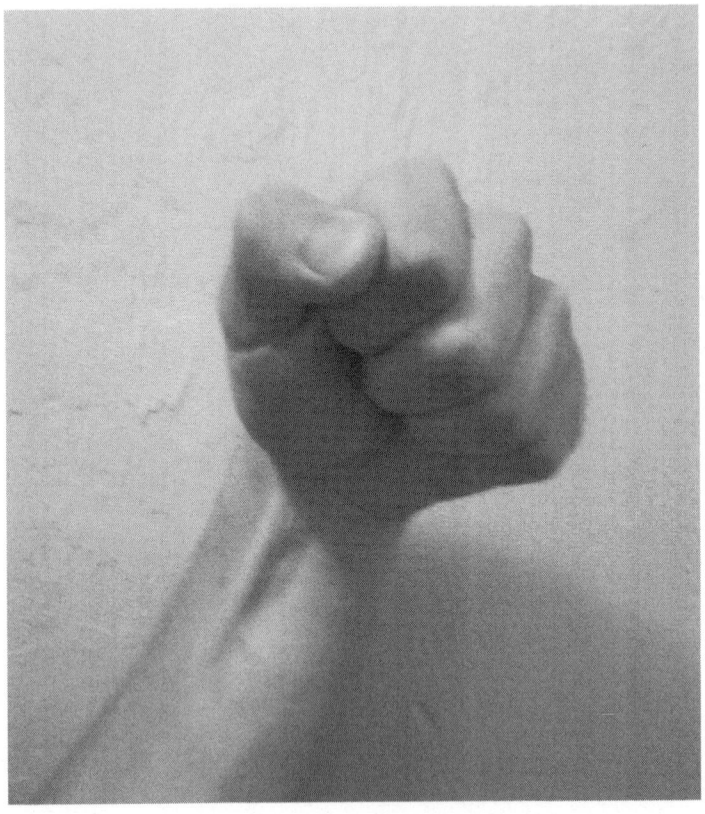

Position 8

Finally, you're going to open your hand as wide as you possibly can, as you did in position 6, but this time you will flex your wrist back as far as you can at the same time.

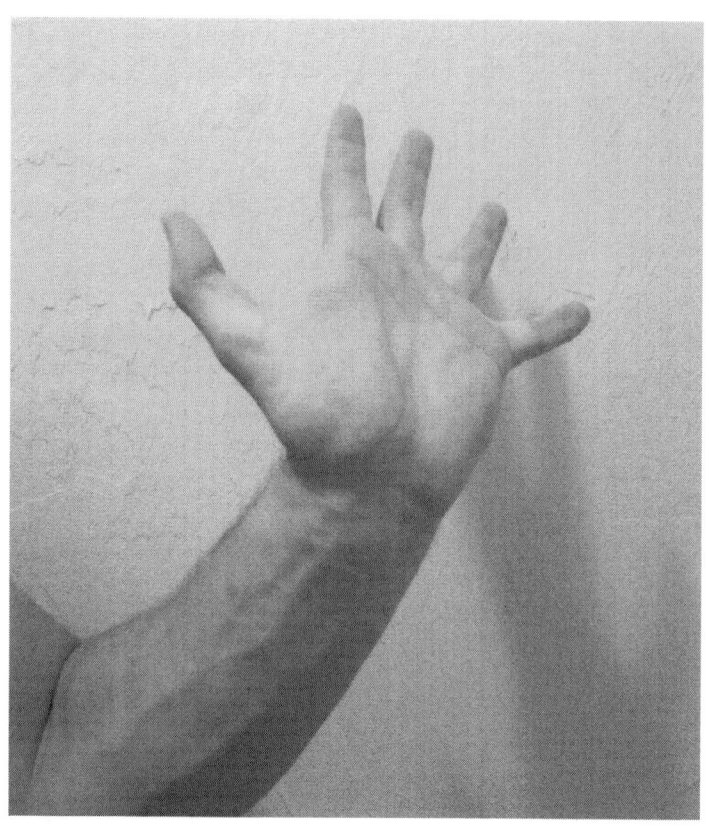

If you've got a morning commute on a bus or train (don't do this while driving, of course), a daily walk, or any other time when your hands are free and you've got a couple of minutes, this is a great way for you to build your hand strength.

At first you probably want to do one hand at a time, because you really get a lot of improvement out of focusing on each specific movement to feel where and how to apply pressure, not to mention training yourself to apply continuous, intense pressure throughout the full ten seconds (this is absolutely key and takes some practice).

Once you're better at that, though, you can do both hands simultaneously. Just remember always to use good form, which means both holding your hands in the correct position as well as applying correct, constant, intense pressure.

Don't underestimate this little routine—doing this alone on a regular basis, even if you don't do anything else in this book, will give you great results and near-complete hand training.

As always, take baby steps in the beginning—it's not too likely that you'd hurt yourself doing isometrics, but if it's your very first attempt, maybe do a 'dry run' of just going through each position and holding with less tension for less time. Then, when you're comfortable, do it for real.

BLOCK WEIGHTS

The block weight is an absolutely fantastic tool for building hand strength. If you can only buy one piece of equipment for grip strength training, make it this.

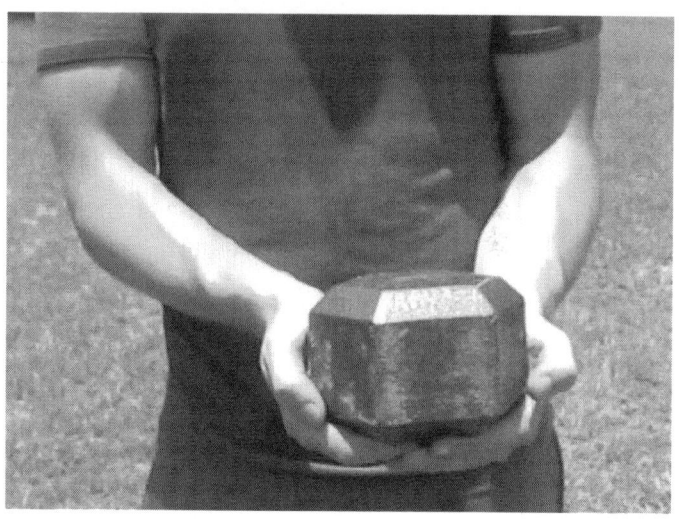

I'm not aware of anyplace where you can buy a block weight directly. As far as I know, you need to make it yourself; we'll talk about that at the end of this chapter.

The block weight is great because it's so simple; it's a heavy object that's difficult to hold, so any simple exercise or lift you do with it develops big-time hand strength.

It also allows for a number of different ways to pick it up, which means you can introduce some variation and do more complete training.

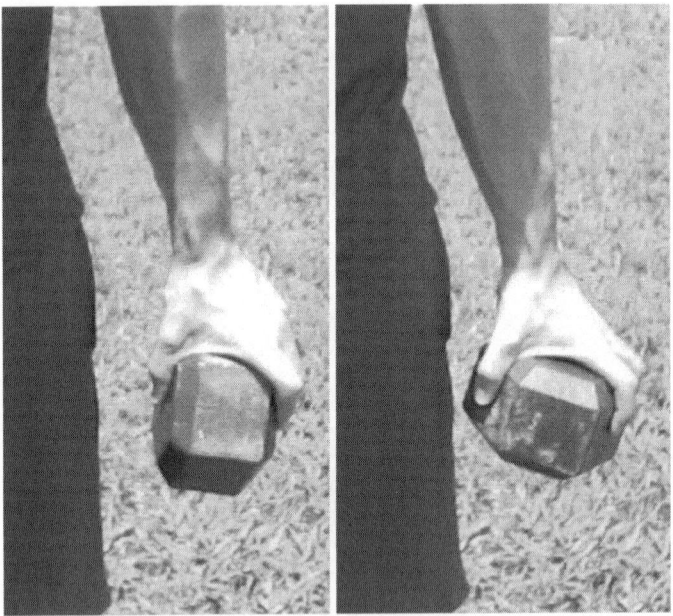

Perhaps the most basic way to train with a block weight is just a simple lift or hold.

Brace the non-lifting arm on your upper leg, bend down, and lift up the weight.

Hand And Forearm Exercises

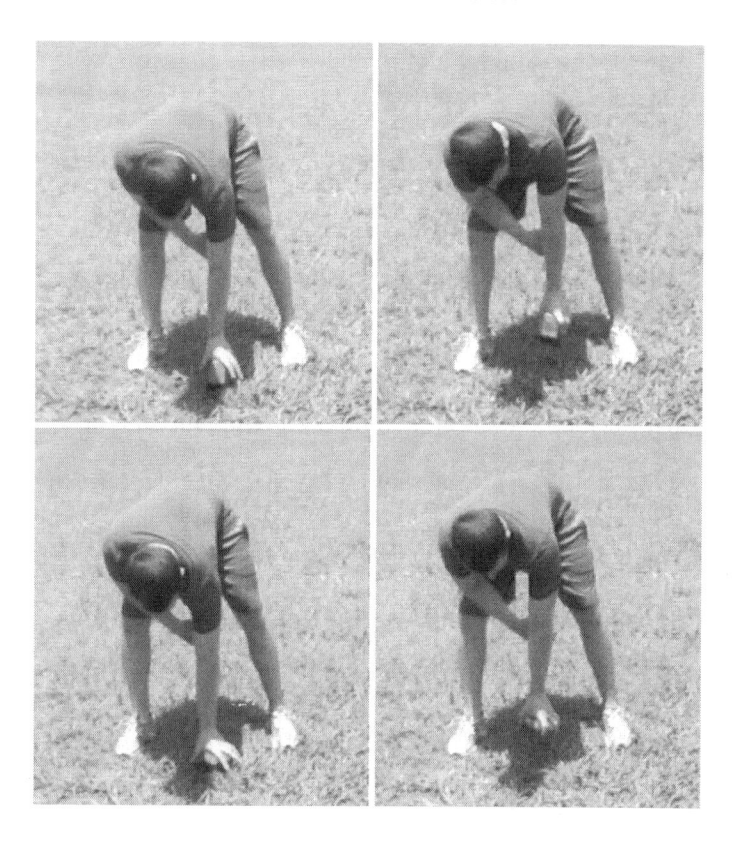

There are two basic approaches for this kind of training: either lift the weight, then put it down again and release your grip, then regrip and lift and repeat until failure (until you can no longer grip the weight to pick it up), or you can simply pick up the weight and hold it until failure. You can also mix and match these techniques.

After doing a set on each hand, go back to the first hand. Since your first hand rested while the second lifted, it should be ready to do another set until failure of either lifts or a hold. Continue sets to failure until you can no longer do the exercise correctly; if that takes a long time then think about getting heavier block weights.

Be sure that whatever you do on one hand, you balance out on the other hand (if you go to failure on one hand, go to failure on the other, and so on.

Another great aspect of block weights is that you can use them to add a new level of difficulty to a variety of other simple dumbbell-type exercises. Here are a few worth trying:

Upright Row

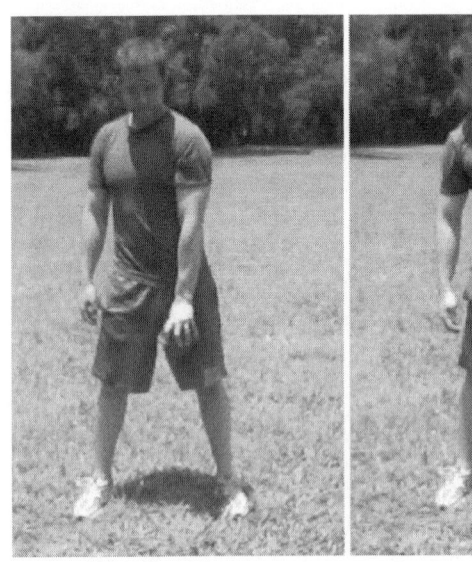

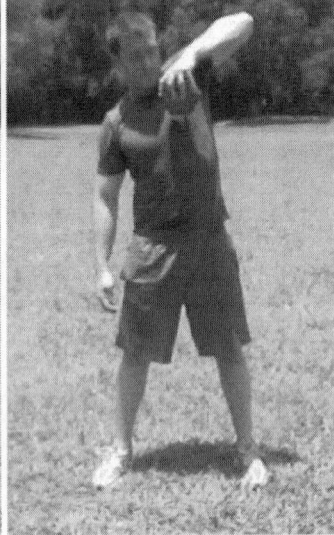

Bent Over Row

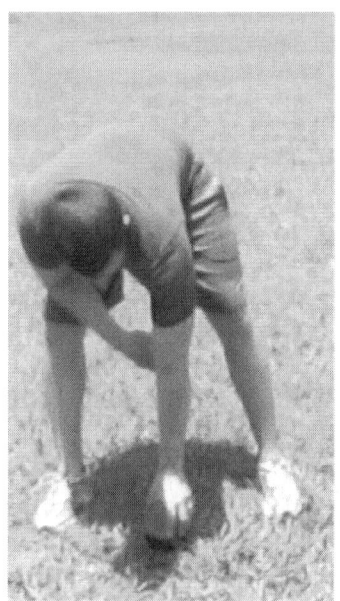

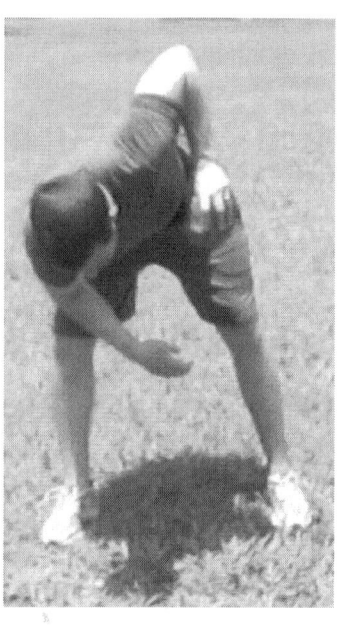

Hammer Curl

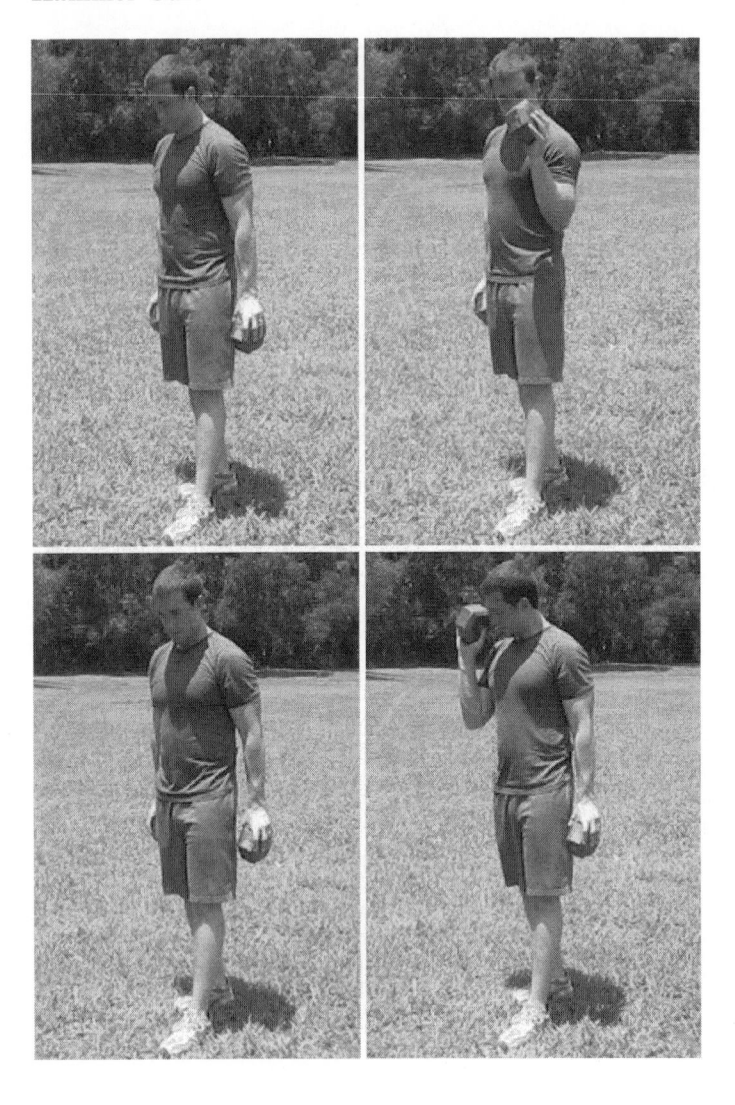

Hand And Forearm Exercises

One-Arm Snatch

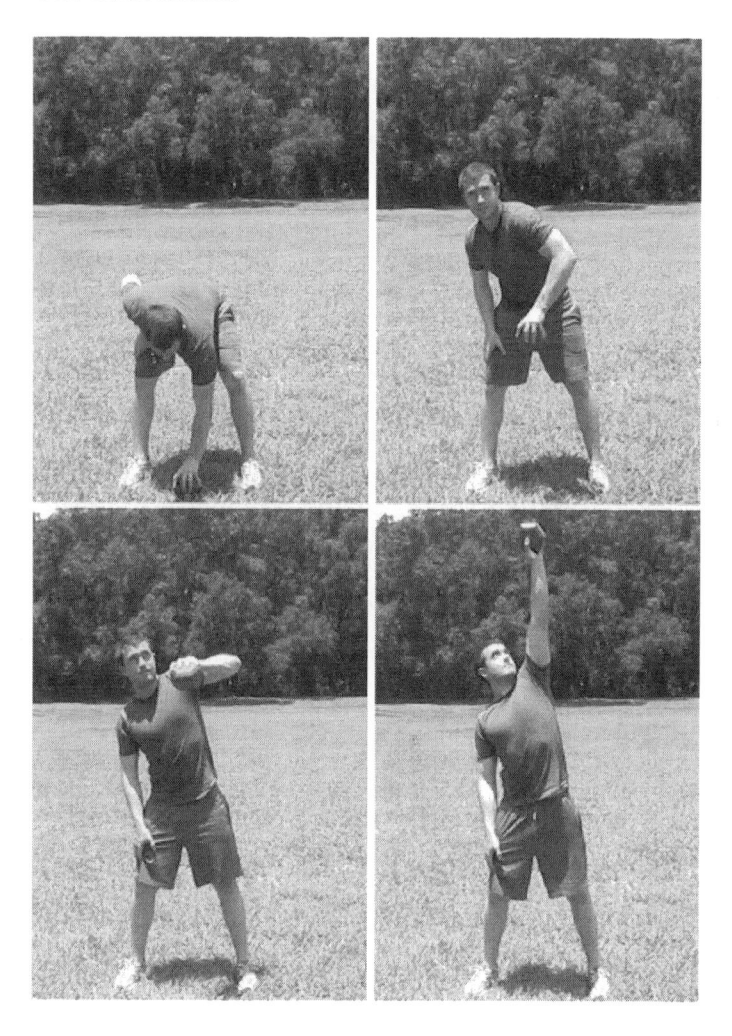

One-Arm Deadlift

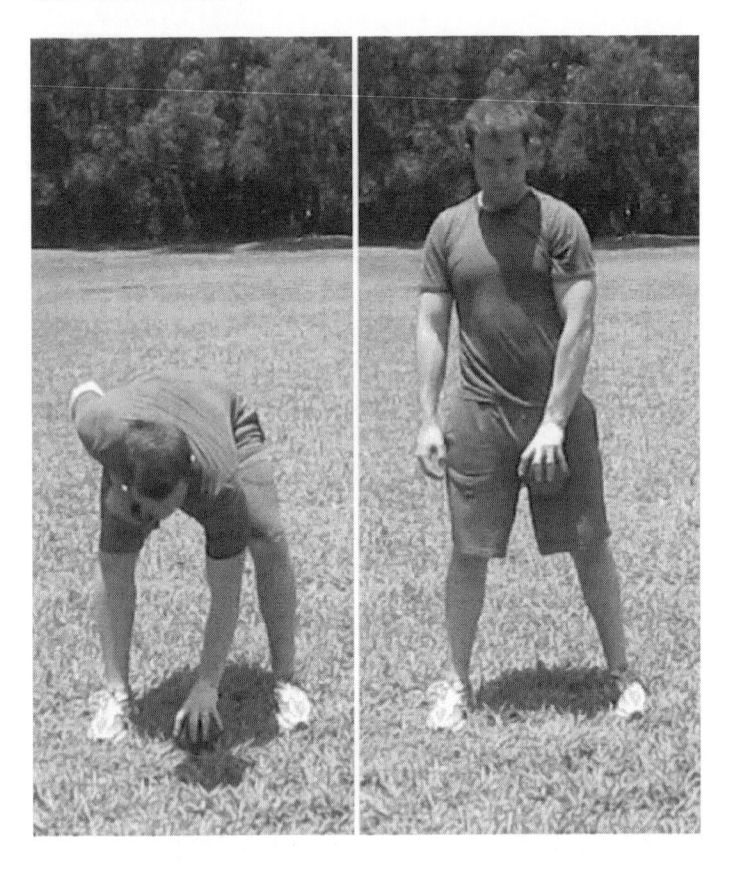

Feel free to try other exercises with block weights, but be sure only to use to do exercises in which you are confident you can control the weight at all times, and which, if you lost control, would not result in the weight falling and injuring you or another person.

Feel free to try other exercises with block weights, but be sure only to use exercises in which you are confident you can control the weight at all times, and which, if you lost control, would not result in the weight falling and injuring you or another person.

Also, be aware that for real benefit, any exercise you do with block weights should have your fingertips pointing downward for some or all of the movement, otherwise you aren't really getting the benefit of gripping the weight.

John Brookfield, who has been able to develop one of the strongest grips of all time, is a huge proponent of block weights (if you're really into grip strength, you should definitely pick up his books).

So now you know that block weights are great. How do you get some of your own?

The only way I know to get them is to make them, and the only way I know to make them is to buy a hex dumbbell—like this one:

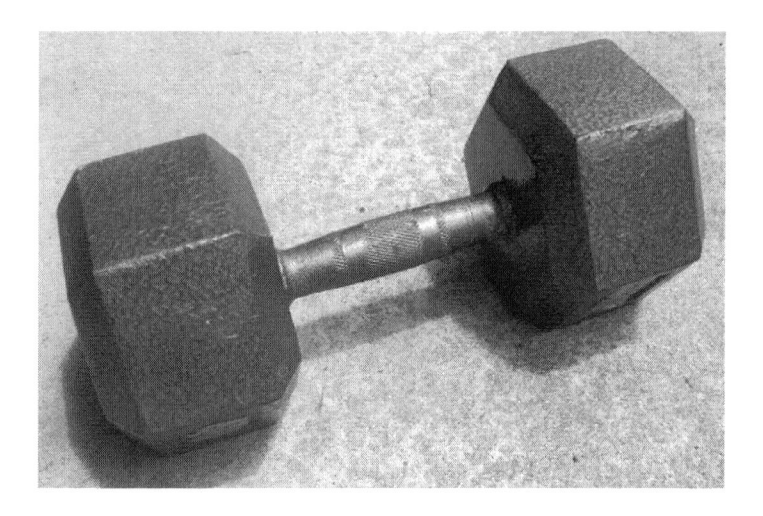

Then, get a hacksaw—

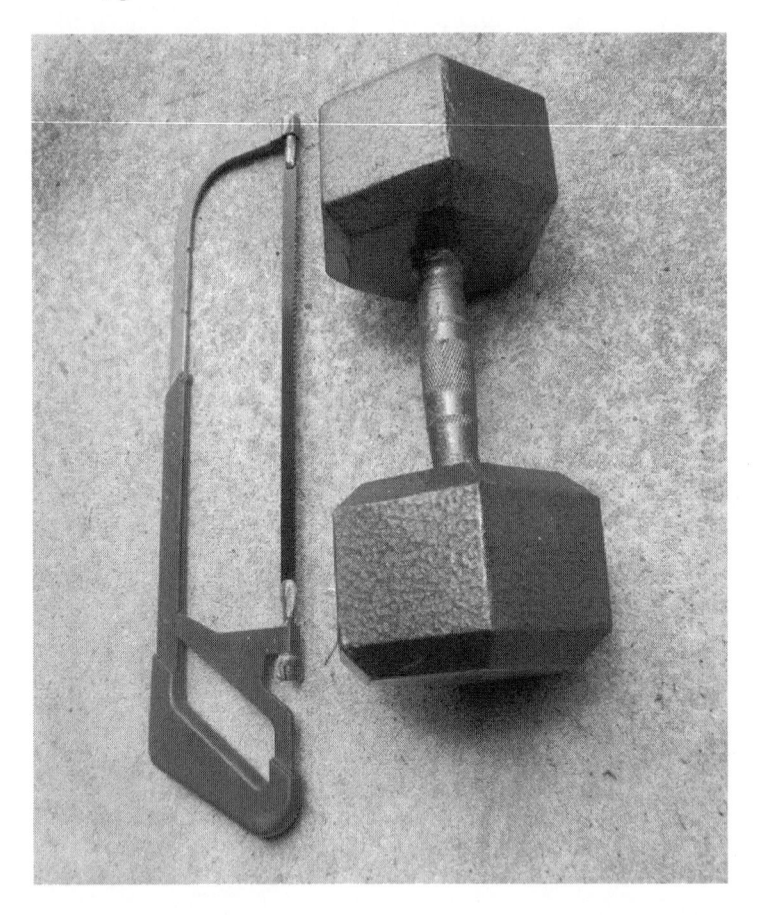

And cut the handle off, as close to the block on the end as possible.

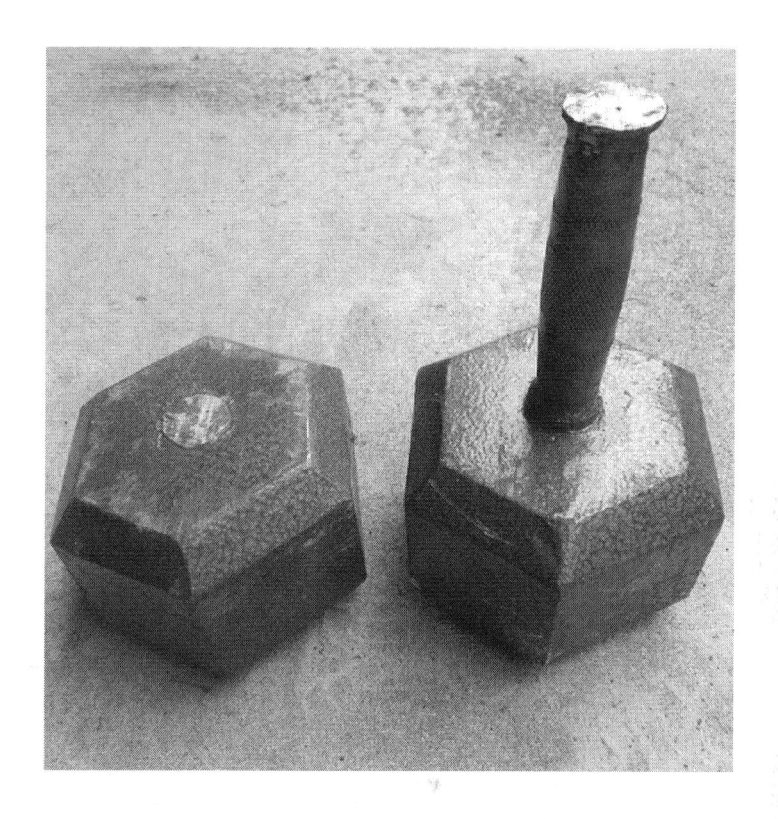

As you might imagine, cutting them off is itself quite a workout. Expect to run through more than one hacksaw blade.

For a reasonably strong person, a good start is a 40 pound dumbbell (which will yield two block weights at just under 20 pounds each). You can go pretty far just using these, but feel free to add heavier weights to your collection to change up the difficulty.

Another Option

The one decent alternative that I've found to block weights is buying pavers from a home improvement store. There's a lot of variability in the thickness and weight of pavers, and depending on where you drop them they might break, but I've found more than a few that do the job quite well.

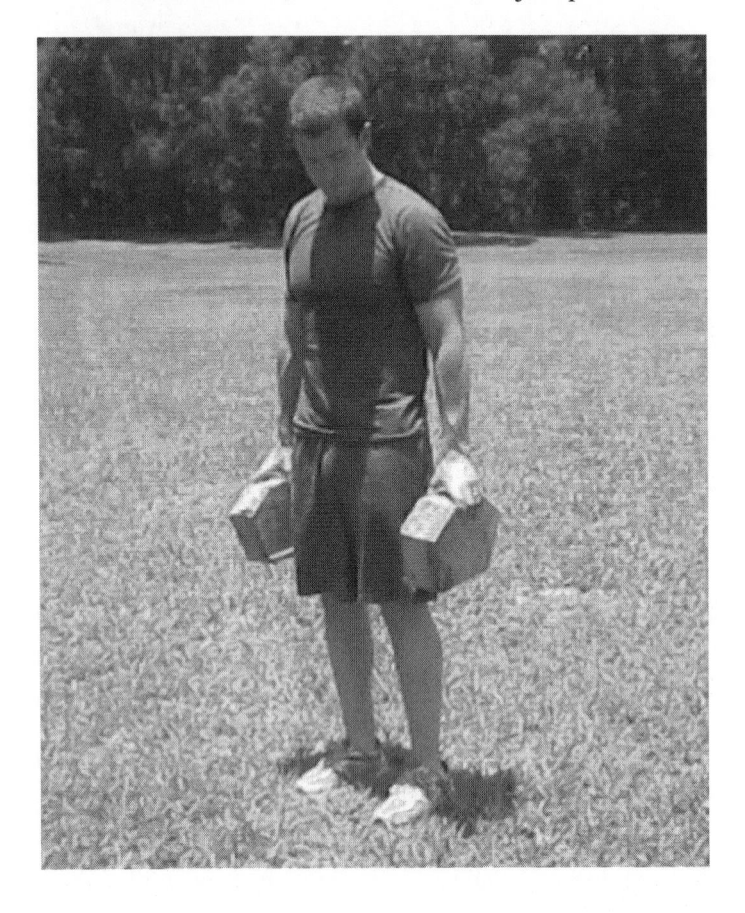

Find the pavers in the store, and pick a few up to see how they feel. Make sure you don't have to open your hands wider than what feels comfortable to grip them, and I would recommend using them outside your house or in your garage. Be sure to find ones that don't have any kind of a raised edge or anything that makes it too easy to grip them.

Pavers are easier to find, you don't need a hacksaw, and they're usually pretty cheap, so you might prefer these to block weights for the sake of convenience.

WALKING BROOM

This is an awesome and simple exercise to increase hand strength and manual dexterity, not to mention shoulder strength.

Simply grab a broomstick in one hand, by the top, and extend your arm straight out to the side or in front of you. Then, keeping your hand steady at the same height, use your fingers to "walk" down the broom, lifting it all the way up until your hand is at the bottom.

Then, "walk" your fingers back up the broom, and return it to its original position.

You'll find that the higher the broom goes, the more difficult it is to keep it under control, and the more challenging the exercise will be. For an added challenge, you can find a heavier broom, or you can even invert it so that the broom head is on top, which makes balancing the broom during the exercise more challenging.

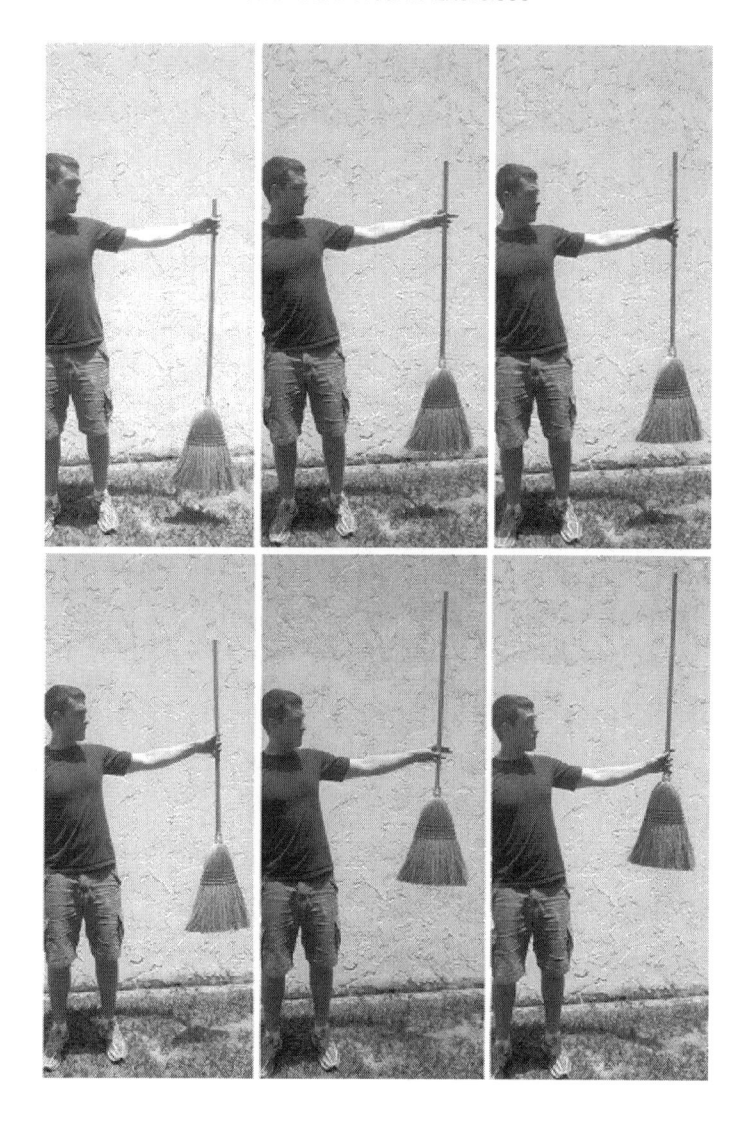

Lowering the broom is much easier than raising it, but you should still take the time to do it correctly to work your fingers in the opposite direction—and you'll find even lowering it gets hard after a few repetitions of going up and down.

Start with one hand first, and using this technique raise the broom all the way up until you are holding it by the bottom end, then walk it back to the position it was in at the beginning. At first one trip might be a good workout, but if not repeat the action until you can no longer do it in good form. Then, switch to the other hand and do the same.

If you don't want to do so many repetitions, increase the difficulty as mentioned before, with a heavier broom, or an inverted broom.

This is a great—and convenient—exercise, so give it a shot.

SLEDGEHAMMER

The sledgehammer is another awesome tool for building wrist and grip strength, not to mention general shoulder and upper body strength. The first exercise we look at will be the sledgehammer tilt, where you tilt the sledgehammer behind your head. Your goal is to be able to lower the sledgehammer until the head of the hammer is behind your head, and then bring it back up to the starting position.

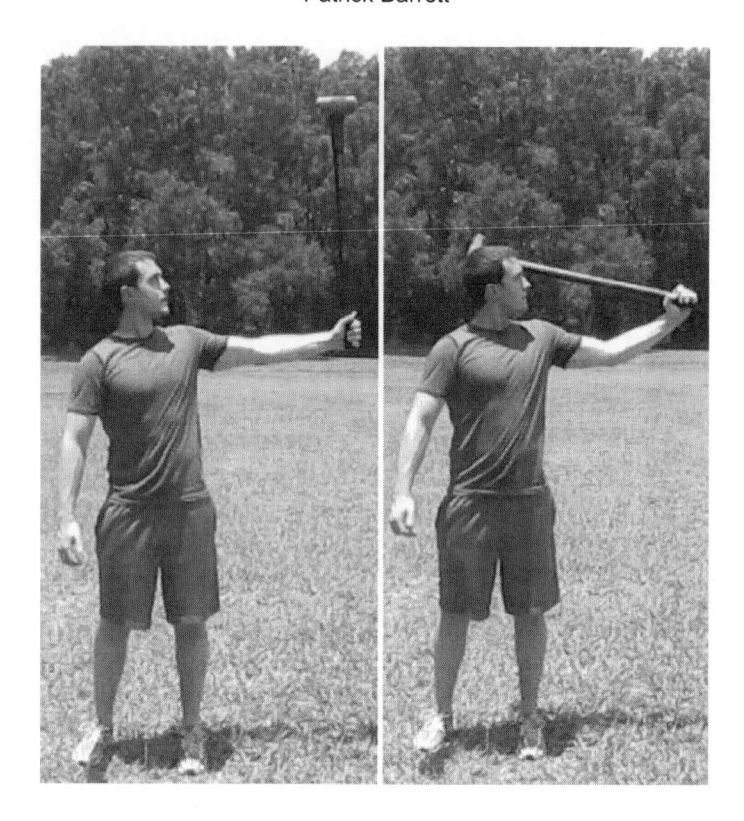

Of course, you need to be very careful here, because you could lose control of the sledgehammer and hurt yourself.

Don't do that. Lower the sledgehammer as far as you can while still controlling it, and then lift it back to the starting position.

At the beginning this may be a very small range of motion; just make sure you stay in control and be patient and you'll make progress. Repeat for 5-10 reps or so.

If you ever lose control of the sledgehammer with one hand, bring your other hand up to stop it.

Hand And Forearm Exercises

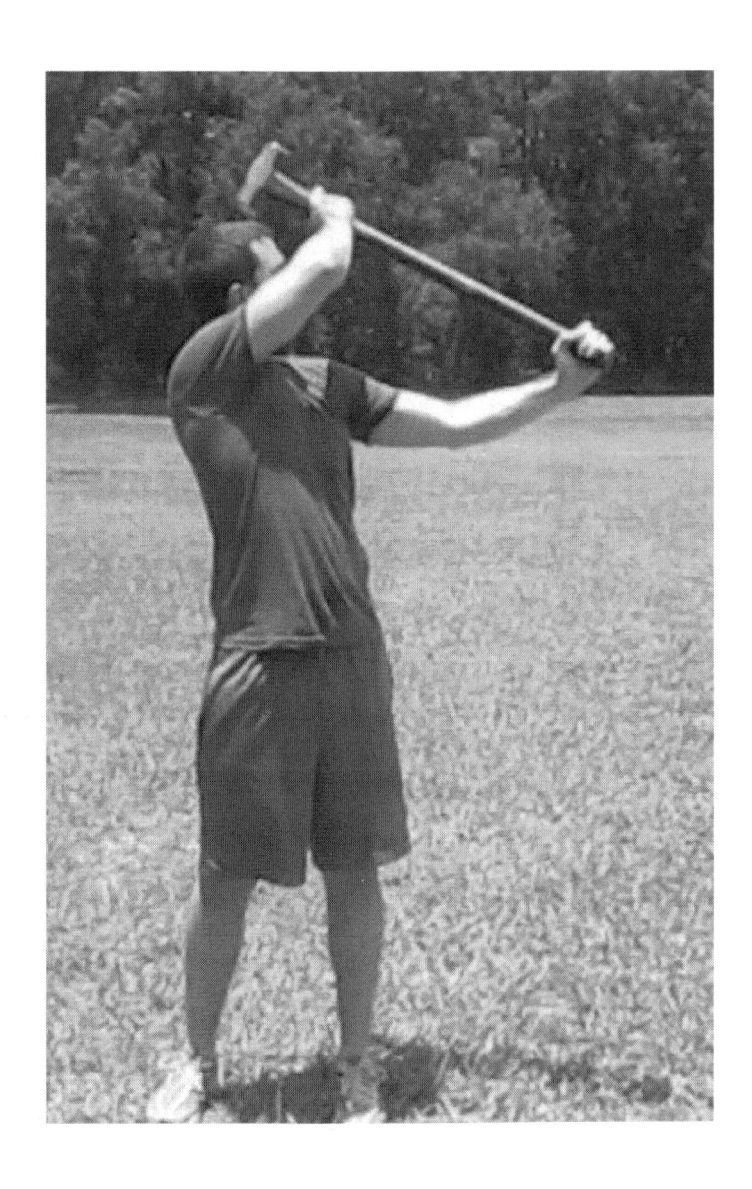

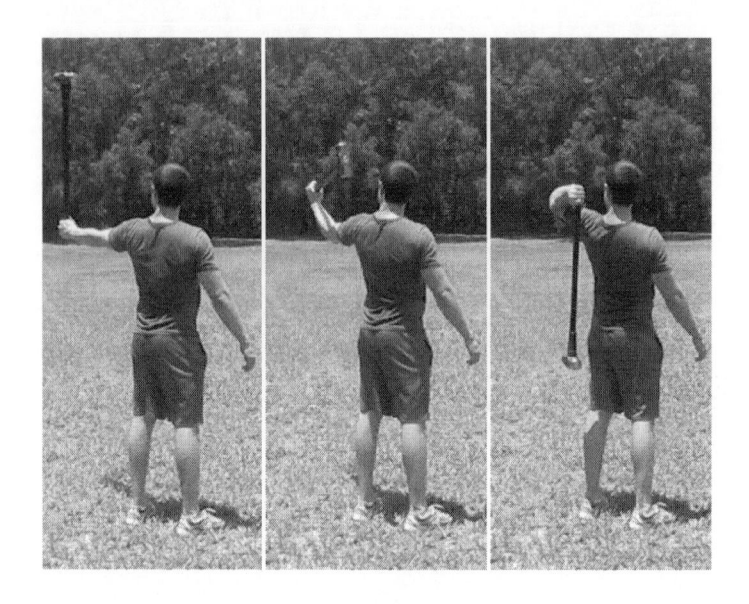

You can also just let the sledgehammer come down behind you without causing any trouble.

Never lower the hammer directly above your head, because the head of the hammer could come down and hit you. Always lower it at an angle behind your head, so if it drops, it drops behind you.

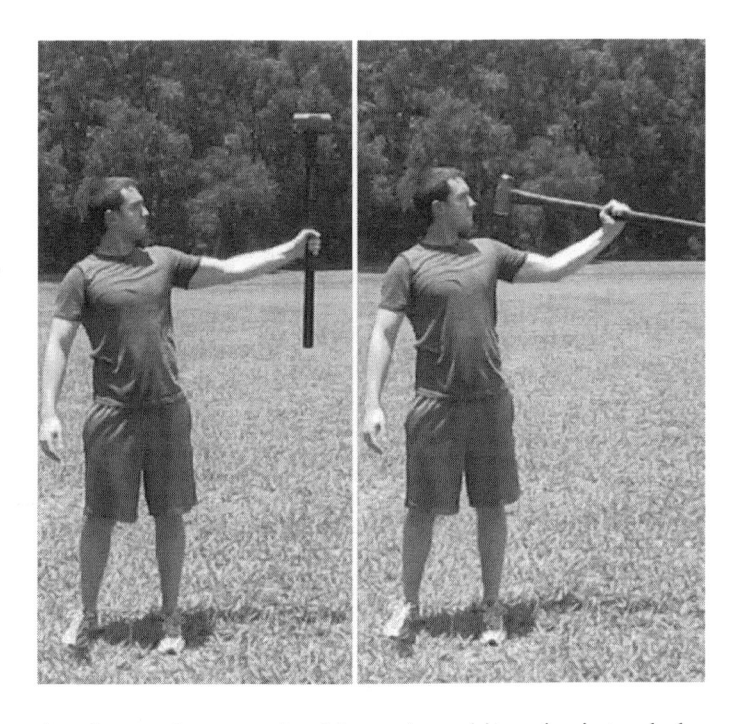

Another option to make this motion a bit easier is to choke up on the hammer; the more you choke up the easier it will be to control it.

The other exercise you'll do is the sledgehammer rotation.

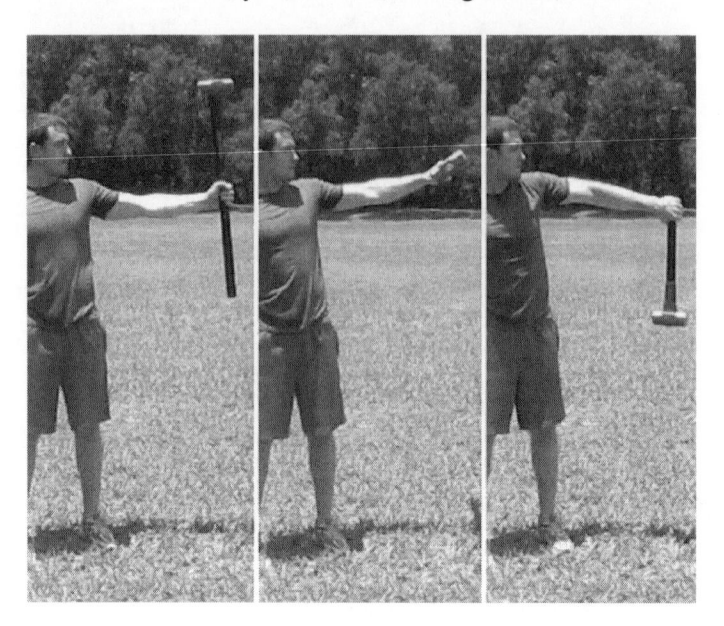

As you can see, you will want to choke up when you do this exercise. I don't want you to wreck anything in your hand, wrist, elbow, shoulder, or anywhere else, so be sure to choke up a lot when you first try any sledgehammer exercise, and only increase the difficulty as you feel comfortable. The next picture shows the rotation with the grip choked up almost all the way to the head of the hammer.

Hold the hammer straight out to your side, or out in front of you, with the head up. In a smooth and controlled motion, rotate your wrist forward so that the hammer goes horizontal, and then is upside down. Then, rotate it back up to the starting position.

This will be hard. Make sure you choke up.

Hand And Forearm Exercises

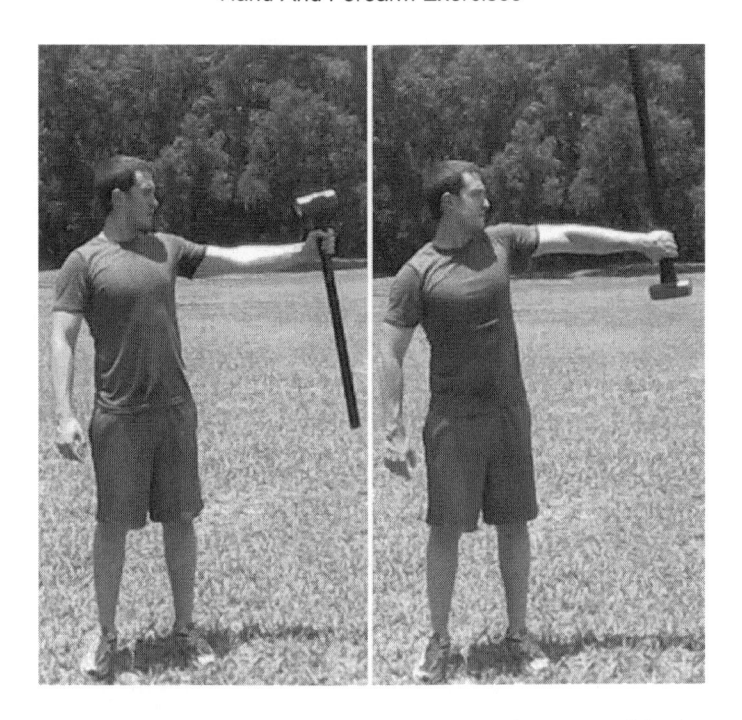

When you do these sledgehammer exercises, as with the block weight exercises or any other exercises in this book, always be sure to think ahead, and don't put yourself in a position where you might injure yourself or someone else. Don't do anything if you think you might lose control of the weight at any point, and think ahead of what to do in case you do lose control.

You can make any sledgehammer exercise easier by gripping the hammer closer to the head. If you're ever unsure of yourself, start by gripping the hammer very close to the head, and only move away a little at a time once you know you can handle it.

Start with something you know you can handle, and then work your way up to something more challenging, but always stay in control.

HANGING

This sounds pretty simple, even stupid, but it's still a worthwhile exercise. Just hang from a bar.

Jump on to the bar, grab on, and hang for as long as you can. Do it for just a little while as part of a warm up, or do it near the end of a workout for as long as you can just to push your endurance to the limit.

You can also take a deep breath, and squeeze extra hard for ten seconds or so, while hanging, as you exhale slowly. Then relax your hands a little (though keep them tight enough so you stay on the bar), take a deep breath, and squeeze hard again during another slow exhale, and so on. This can really do a lot to work your grip and your forearms.

Hand And Forearm Exercises

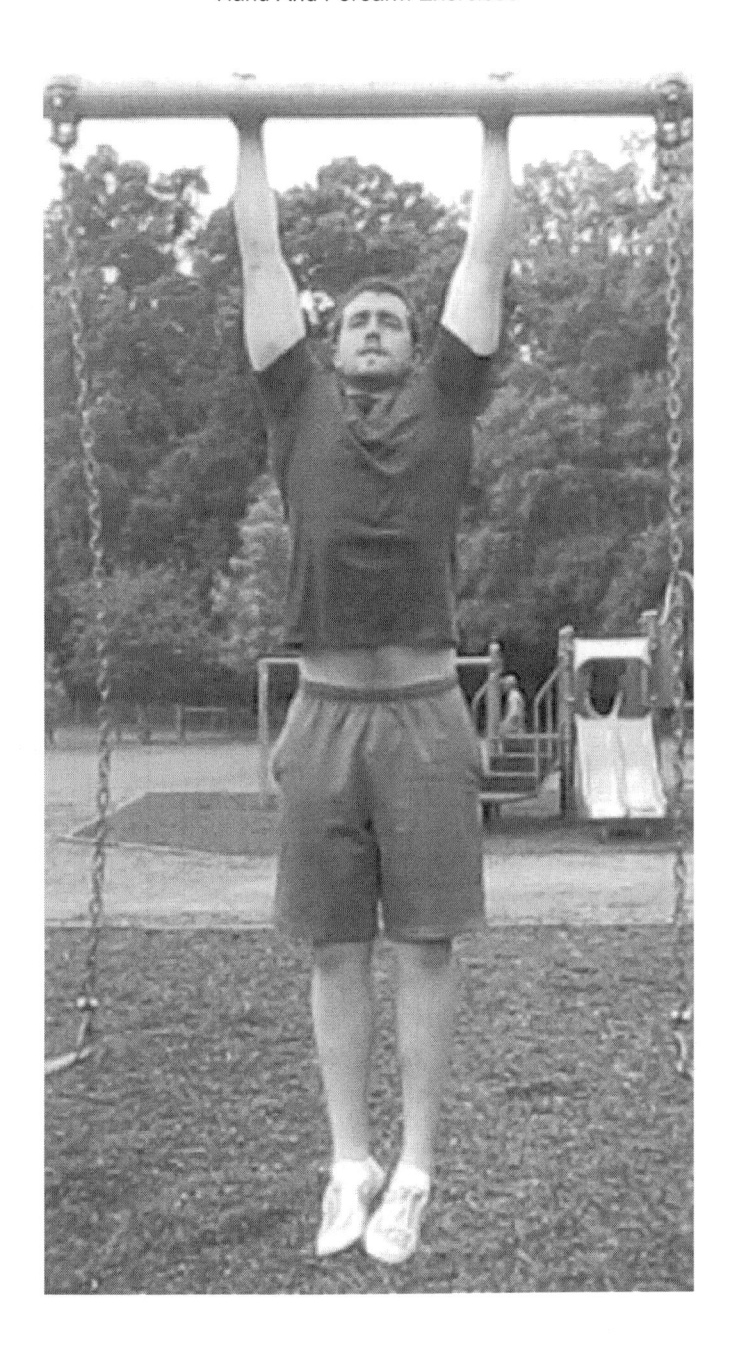

FARMER'S CARRY

This is another simple exercise, but it can be extremely effective in building strength in your hands and forearms, as well as your shoulders.

Just find two similar heavy objects, pick one up in each hand, and walk as far as you can.

These can be dumbbells, kettlebells, block weights, jugs filled with water or sand, or, as in the picture, you can do them carrying pavers. Just make sure they're both the same weight for the sake of balance, then pick them up and walk as far as you can.

When you can't hold them any longer, stop walking and put them down. Take a few breaths and a rest for 30 seconds or a minute, then pick them back up and keep walking again. Repeat until you're too fatigued to continue.

Hand And Forearm Exercises

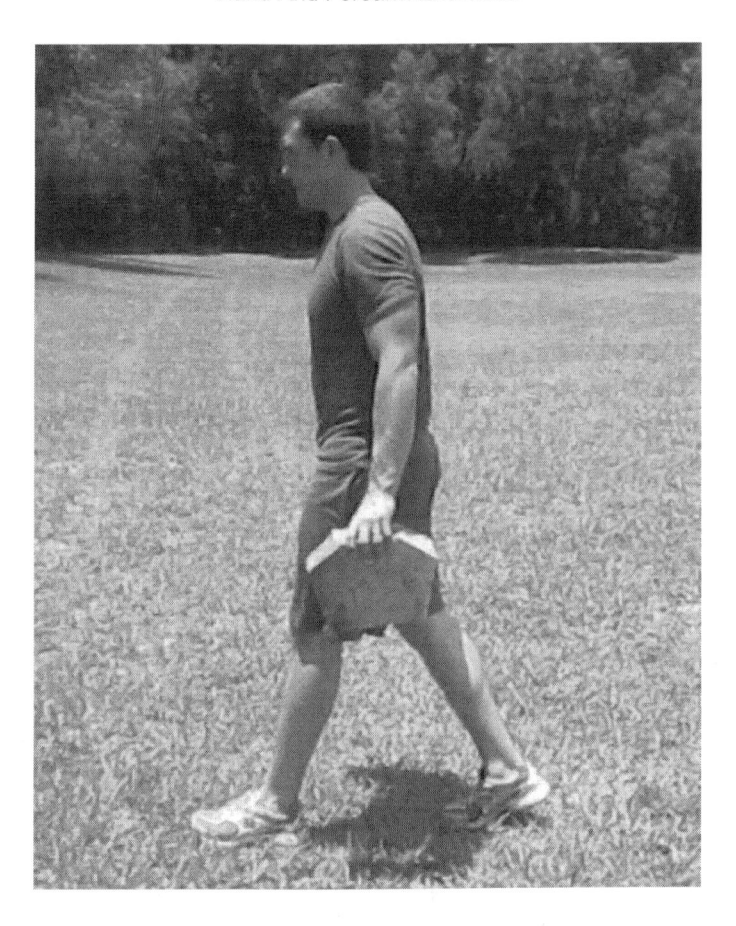

You probably want to follow some kind of route or pattern when you walk, and bear in mind that when you're done you've got to bring your weights back to where you started, so you might not want to end up too far away.

GYRO BALL

These are awesome. I'm not big on training gadgets in general, but this is a definite exception. I love playing with this thing; it takes a little time to get the hang of it, but it's worth it.

The basic idea is that you grip the outer housing of the gyro ball in your hand. Inside is basically a weighted wheel which can spin in all directions. Once you start the spin, and you get your technique down, you'll be able to feel the force generated as the inner wheel spins at thousands of RPMs. Believe it or not, those RPMs produce (in the standard models) around 30 lbs of force.

It's hard to describe the feeling you have when you use one of these balls, but try to imagine holding onto a billiard ball that's trying to fight its way out of your hand using 30 pounds of force that is constantly changing directions.

See? Hard to describe, and hard to imagine until you've felt it.

Hand And Forearm Exercises

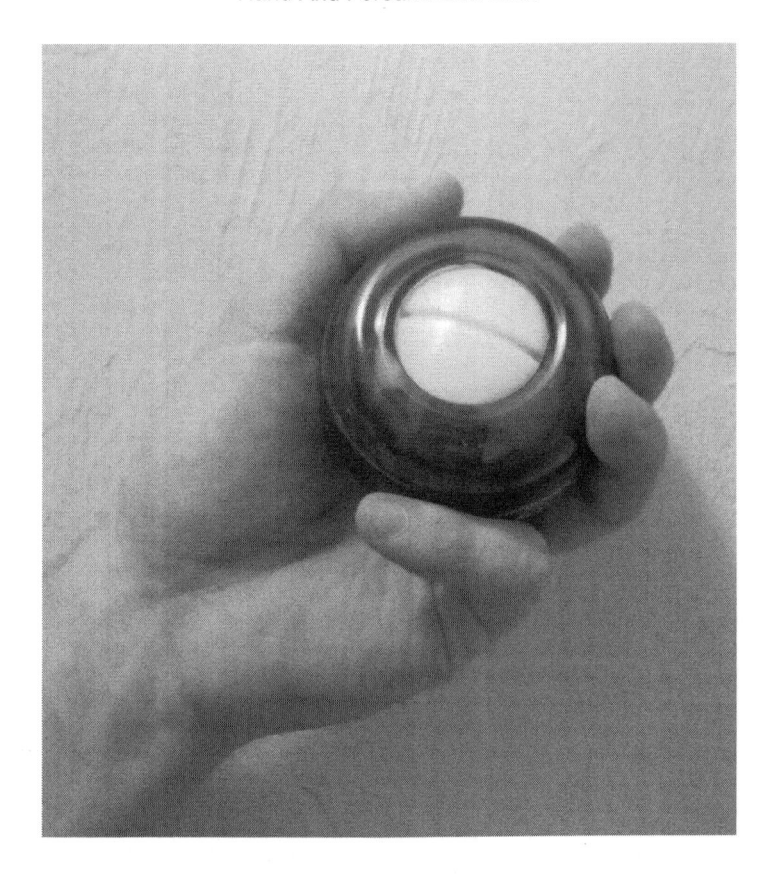

The basic idea is that as the ball fights to go in one direction, you must guide it through another direction. If it's trying to rotate clockwise, you grip it and rotate it counter-clockwise, and so on. This will keep the wheel spinning faster and faster, increase the torque, and give you a great forearm workout.

The bottom line here is that you need to use one of these to understand what a great tool it is. If you're at all interested in this idea, I encourage you to order one and give it a shot. Here are some tips you can put into use if you decide to get one.

******

At first, your goal with the gyro ball is just to get it going. It should come with a string and instructions on how to get it started. Follow these, at least in the beginning, because the string is the most surefire way to get the ball going.

Once you've used the ball, you have an idea for the kind of technique you need to get it going. That's very important if you want to learn to start the ball without the string, which is much more convenient. There are a few methods for starting the ball without the string. Here's my favorite.

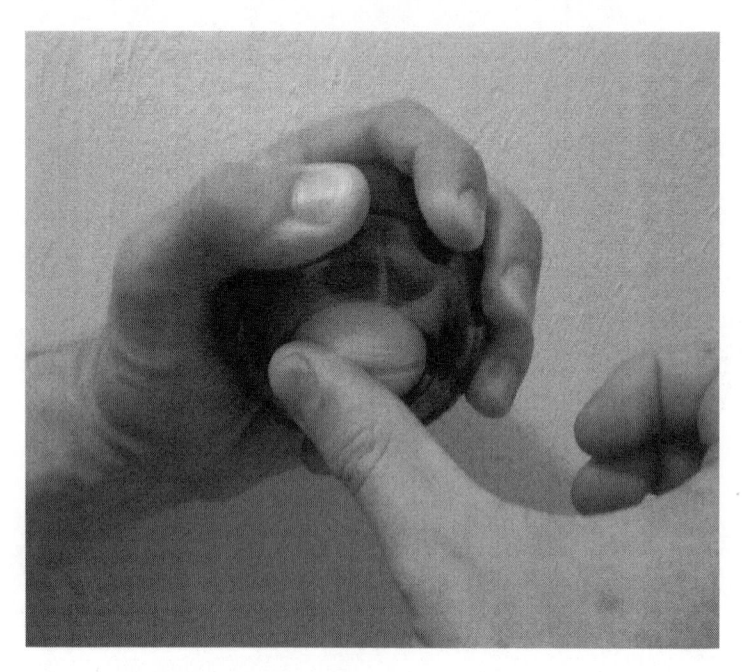

Hand And Forearm Exercises

Hold the ball as pictured. Note that the wheel will roll in the direction of the line across the middle of the wheel. Press your thumb toward the center of the ball from the position pictured. Then, slide your thumb forward hard so that the wheel begins to spin rapidly.

At this point, the wheel should be spinning reasonably fast, but not fast enough yet to get started. Immediately after you spin the wheel, begin rotating the ball like this.

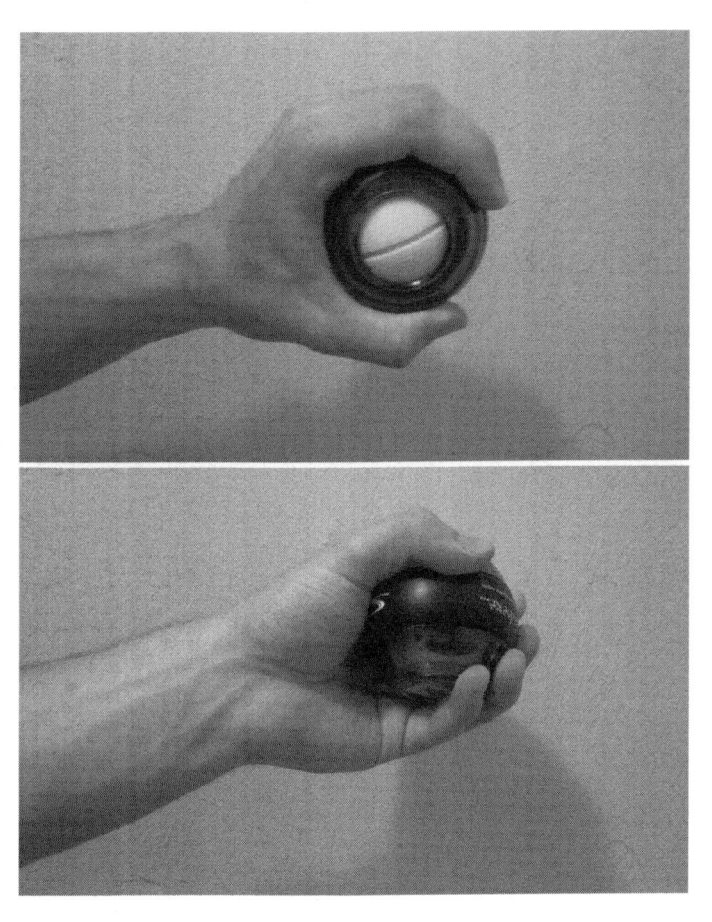

Grip the ball and rotate it left, then right, almost the way you would turn a doorknob. If it's working, you should start to feel some of the forces you felt when you started it with the string, and you should be set. If not, repeat the process.

The first time you start the ball in this way might take a while, but afterward you will get the hang of it.

Once you are used to starting the ball, you can start working out with it. There are three basic ways to move the ball that I like to use. The first is the easiest, and it's the one we just talked about using to get the ball started. Simply hold the ball as shown in the previous pictures, and rotate left, then right, like a doorknob.

The next variation is harder.

Hold the ball with your palm against the back of the ball, as shown. Rotate your wrist in a full circle, to the back, down, to the front, up, and so on. Once you get the ball started and then try this motion, you'll feel the right path to follow. You can also reverse the path and rotate in the other direction for a more complete workout.

This is a reasonably challenging movement, and it can give you a great forearm and hand workout.

Hand And Forearm Exercises

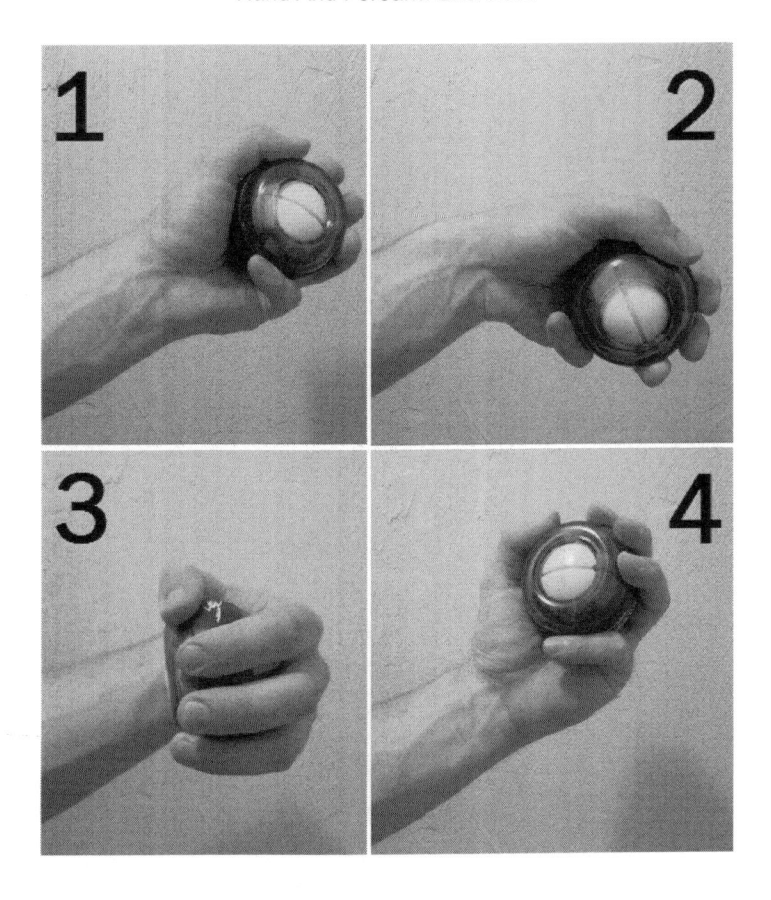

This brings us to the third and most difficult variation.

As you can see, in this variation you hold the ball with your fingertips. Then, follow the same path as you did in the last sequence, rotating your wrist in a full circle, to the back, down, to the front, up, and so on.

This is a difficult movement, and will really help develop powerful strength in your forearm and fingers.

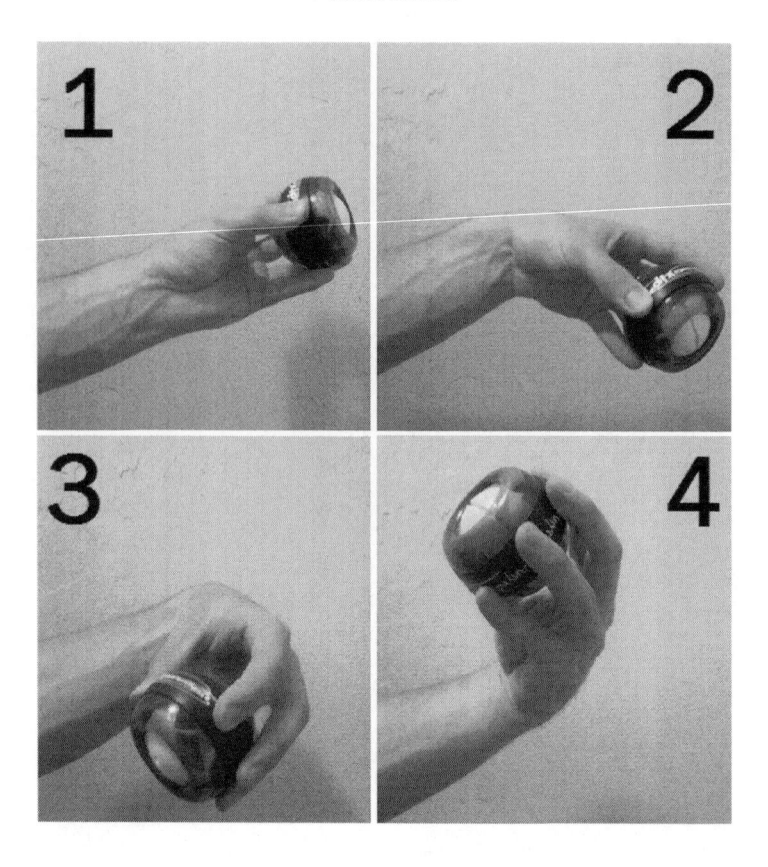

Bear in mind that you shouldn't attempt this unless you feel reasonably confident in your ability to hold onto the ball. Even so, you may want to attempt it while sitting on a carpeted floor, or over a bed or couch, so that if you drop the ball you don't damage it—dropping the gyro ball onto a hard surface can damage it and cause it not to work properly anymore.

As far as a workout is concerned, I just like to keep the ball going for as long as I can. You can do this while watching TV, taking a walk (be careful not to drop it!) or while doing almost anything else that you don't need your hands for.

I start the ball in one hand, go as long as I can, then I move it to my other hand, and do that for as long as I can. By that point my first hand has rested, so I can switch back to that one and continue, and so on.

You can mix up the grips you use for a more challenging or less challenging workout; using the first motion we discussed (the easier doorknob-turning motion) allows you to rest a little bit and keep the session going.

Keep in mind that you need to practice switching the ball from one hand to another. You'll need to get the ball going fast enough that it won't 'die' and need to be restarted again, but not so fast that you can't control it (experiment to find the right speed). Once you're there, carefully switch it from the first hand to a solid grip in your other hand.

You need to do this reasonably quickly, but you do have a little bit of time. It won't 'die' right away or anything, you just don't want to take too long. You'll get a feel for it once you've done it a few times.

To make your gyro ball sessions more intense, trying holding the ball with your arm straight out to one side, or straight out in front of you, or straight up above your head. This will engage your shoulders and other muscles in your arm and make the workout even more challenging.

If you don't have one of these balls, this chapter probably didn't make much sense. If this sounds interesting to you, though, you should definitely consider getting one and adding it in to your routine. This is certainly the most enjoyable exercise tool I've ever used, and besides being fun, and a little bit different, it also gives you an impressive grip and forearm workout.

HANDSTANDS

One of the best and simplest ways to develop strong hands is by doing handstands. Many people think that handstand training is primarily for the shoulders and triceps, but the more you do it, the more it strengthens your hands themselves.

To get the full hand-strengthening benefit of doing handstands, you need to be able to hold a free-standing handstand, without the help of a wall. If you can't do that already, learning how to is a project of its own that's too much to cover in this book. You could actually write an entire short book on that subject alone—and I have. If you want to learn how to hold a free handstand, up to and including free standing handstand pushups, you might want to pick up a copy of my book, *How To Do A Handstand*, availabe from Amazon.com and other retailers.

However, even though we aren't going to go through the whole process of learning how to hold a free handstand, we can still talk about doing a supported handstand against a wall, to get you started.

First of all, it should go without saying that you need some upper body strength to do this. The heavier you are, the more you will need. It doesn't require an exceptional level of upper body strength, but I don't want you to get hurt trying something you aren't ready for.

If you can do 10 or 20 pushups in good form, this should be no problem for you. If you think you might not be quite there yet, work on sets of pushups until you are.

Let's start by looking at the sequence.

Start by finding a flat, open area against a wall. Make sure there is nothing nearby that you might knock into or knock over if you run into any trouble.

Get down on all fours facing the wall, with your fingertips about a foot from the wall.

Get into a sort of runner's stance, up on your toes, with one foot just outside the center-line of your body underneath you (this is your trailing foot), and the other just outside the center-line of your body a couple of feet behind the first foot (this is your leading foot).

Lift your leading foot up, and press gently and smoothly off the ground with your trailing foot. It is important to take baby steps here, so just press off a little bit, and then a little bit more, until you are able to gauge the amount of strength you need. Better to jump not hard enough than to jump too hard when you're still learning.

Hand And Forearm Exercises

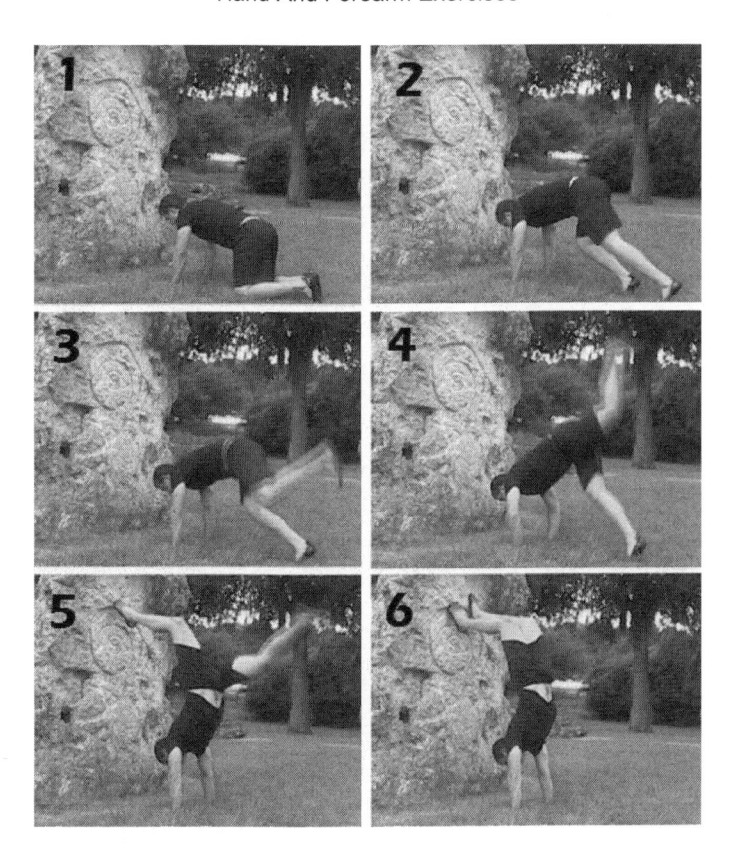

As you press off with your trailing foot, lift your leading foot up toward the wall. As your leading foot moves toward the wall, and 'lands' on the wall, bring up your trailing foot behind it, until both feet are on the wall, and you are holding a supported handstand.

There are two big things you want to keep in mind. The first is not to kick up super hard in the beginning—start with little jumps with your trailing foot and increase the power until you've got enough to kick all the way up. Always stay in control. The second is to make sure that you keep your arms straight and strong and ready to support your weight when you actually get vertical after the kick up.

To get down from the handstand, simply reverse this process. Press against the wall with your leading foot while you bring your trailing foot back down to the floor, with your leading foot following soon after.

At first, just kicking up will be a challenge, and you'll need to work to develop this skill. Instead of spending much time holding the handstand, you're probably better off kicking up into one, holding for just a couple of seconds, then coming back down and kicking up again until you're fatigued.

It shouldn't take long for you to get completely comfortable with kicking up. Then, concentrate on holding the handstand—take deep breaths, stretch your whole body out and try to lengthen your body as much as you can. To increase the difficulty and the work on your hands, do the handstands with your fingertips closer and closer to the wall—the closer they are to the wall, the more your body is directly above your hands and the more you need to use your hands to balance.

Holding these supported handstands for time will strengthen your arms, shoulders, and back. They will also strengthen your hands, especially as your fingertips move closer to the wall. However, for the full hand-strength benefit of this exercise, you really need to learn to do handstands without the help of a wall. If that sounds interesting to you, you might want to check out my full book on the subject, *How To Do A Handstand*, which will teach you how to train to do the free standing handstand in a matter of weeks, and then how to move from there to the free standing handstand pushup.

DUMBBELL TWIST

I feel like I need to include these, since they were the first forearm exercise my dad ever taught me, back when I was in elementary school. It's an oldie but a goodie, and a great option if you're looking for an exercise that just uses standard weights.

As you can see, you're going to stand with your feet shoulder-width apart, holding two dumbbells. Then, twist both dumbbells all the way outward, then all the way inward, then back to the starting position. This is one repetition.

There are two key things to keep in mind in order to get the most out of this exercise. Number one, don't overrotate in either direction, which can cause injury. Twist outward as far as is still comfortable, and do the same on the twist back. Number two, keep in control of the weights. Don't just let them move on momentum; keep a firm grip on the weight and turn smoothly and steadily in one direction, and then smoothly and steadily in the other.

Hand And Forearm Exercises

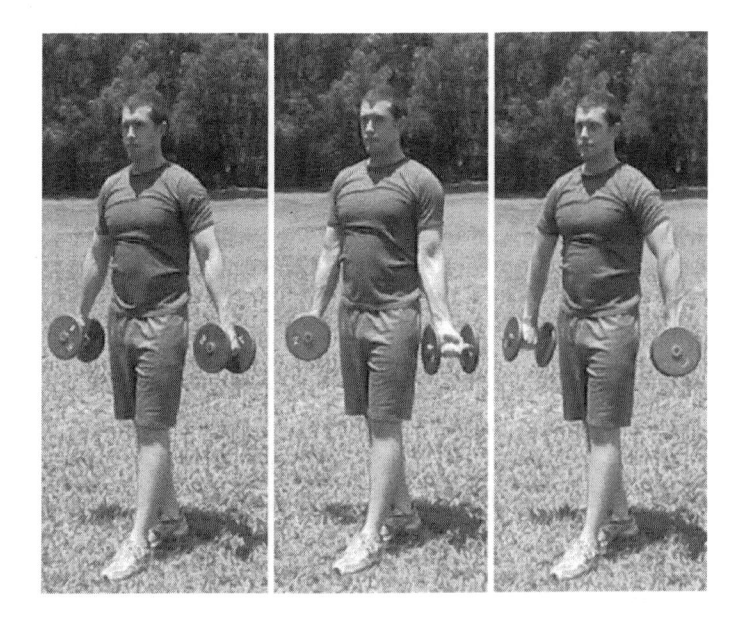

Heavier (and larger) weights can be difficult to rotate in control through a whole range of motion, and they can make it more likely that you will overrotate and injure yourself. Find a weight that you can twist for 20-50 repetitions for a great forearm workout.

FINGERTIP PUSHUPS AND PLANKS

No equipment? No problem. You can take one of the best, simplest exercises and make a small tweak to create an intense hand-strengthening workout session.

First off, fingertip pushups are a classic way to build real hand and finger strength. Take a look at the picture on the next page to see what a standard fingertip pushup looks like.

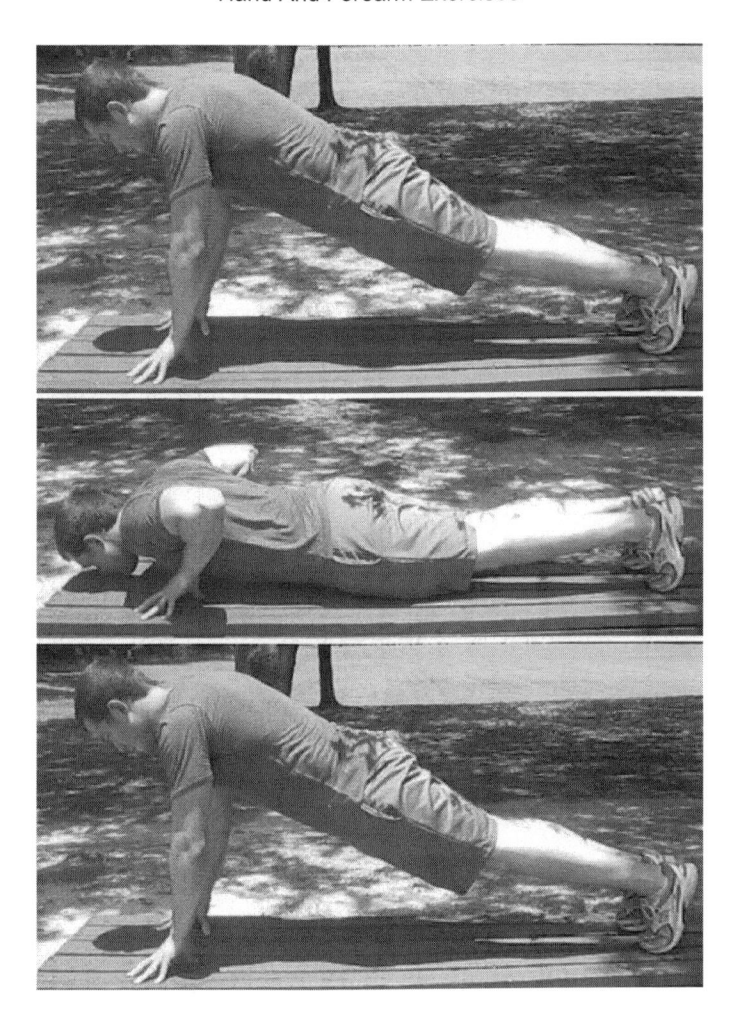

If you're on the heavier side, or if you don't have much experience with this, you might find them to be pretty challenging.

To build up to this skill, just do pushups with one hand in the fingertip pushup position, and the other hand in the normal, flat position. Get in this position, and do one pushup. Then, flatten out the hand in the fingertip position, and put the flat hand in the fingertip position, and do another pushup, then switch back, and so on. Always make sure to do the same number of repetitions focusing on each side.

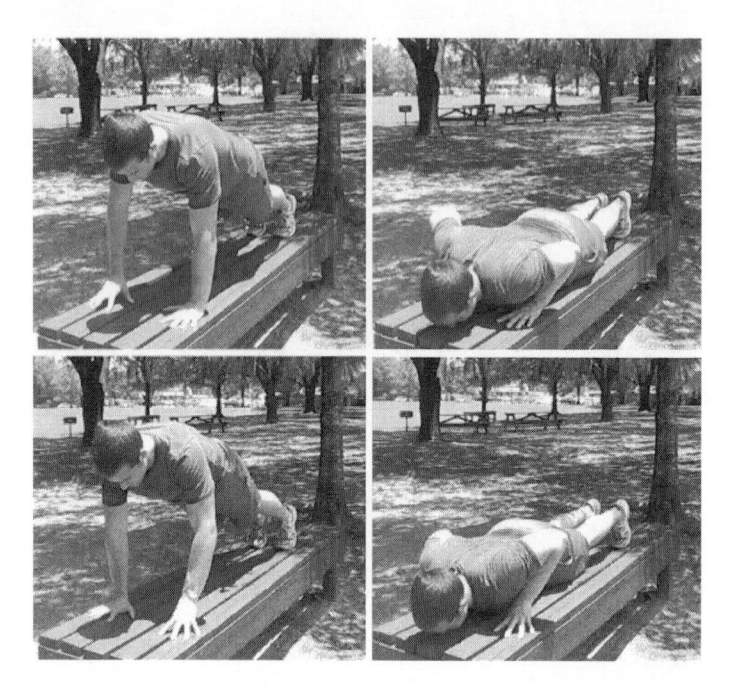

In this way, you can put less stress on your fingers than you would in a normal fingertip pushup while still strengthening them, and before long you'll be able to do normal fingertip pushups.

Another way to get used to doing fingertip pushups (which also happens to be another great exercise on its own) is the fingertip plank.

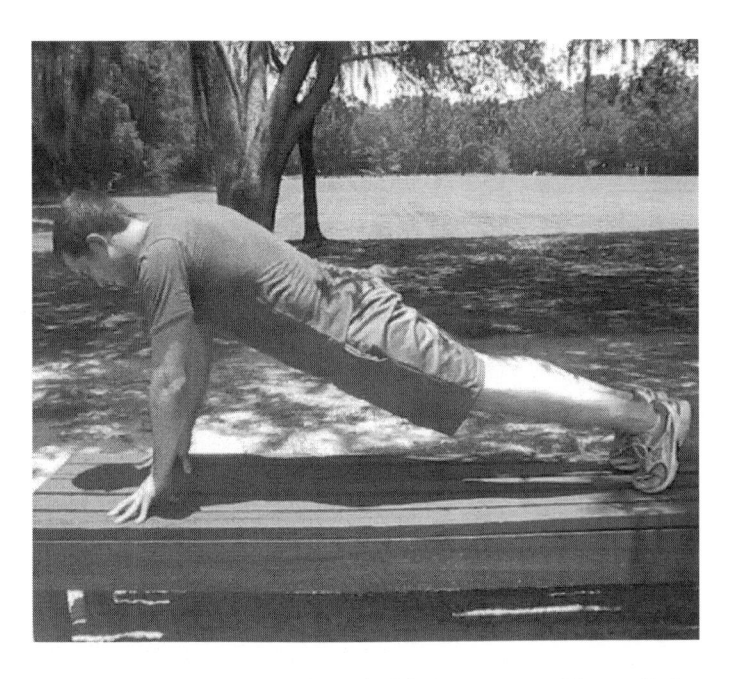

As you can see, you just hold the up position of the fingertip pushup for time. Be sure to use good form, and don't allow your hips to rise too high or drop too low; you should be able flex your abs and feel them supporting the weight of your hips. This doesn't have a huge impact on your fingertip workout, but it will make sure you get a good ab workout at the same time.

All three of these exercises—fingertip pushups, alternating fingertip pushups, and fingertip planks—are wonderful exercises that require no equipment and get great results. Give them a shot, and then add them to your normal routine.

ROPE CLIMBING

This is another simple, amazing exercise that builds upper body strength and serious grip strength. You'll need to start out by finding a rope you can climb.

This is very important—do not climb any rope, or anything else for that matter, that is not securely fastened and capable of supporting at least twice your bodyweight. The last thing you want to do is injure yourself in a fall.

Also, no matter how strong the rope is, do not climb to any height that could result in an injury if you were to lose your grip and fall. Always take every reasonable precaution to make sure you avoid injury when you exercise.

You can start out by just hanging from the rope.

Hand And Forearm Exercises

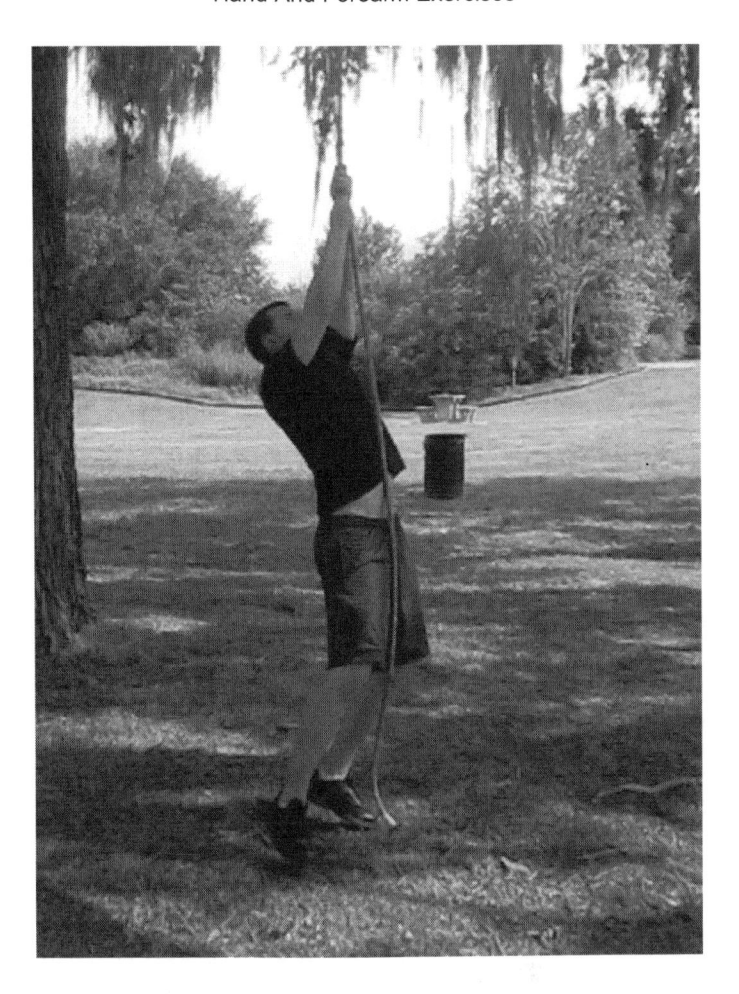

Then, do pull ups on the rope. Alternate which hand is on top, and which hand is on the bottom, and as always do the same number of reps in each position.

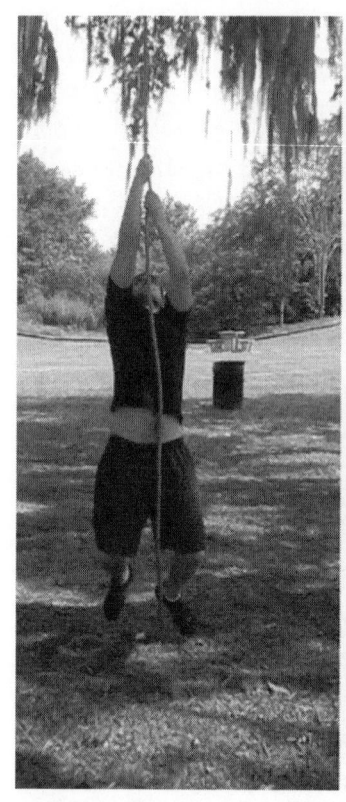

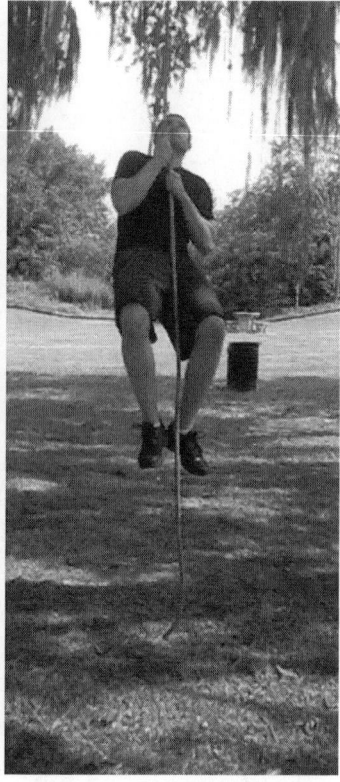

After you can do at least ten rope pull ups, you are ready to start climbing.

Grab on to the rope with both hands. Begin to pull up with both hands. When your top arm is bent at about 90 degrees, reach up with your lower arm and grab the rope about a foot above your other arm. Then pull up again, and when your new top arm is bent at about 90 degrees, reach up with the other arm, and so on.

Hand And Forearm Exercises

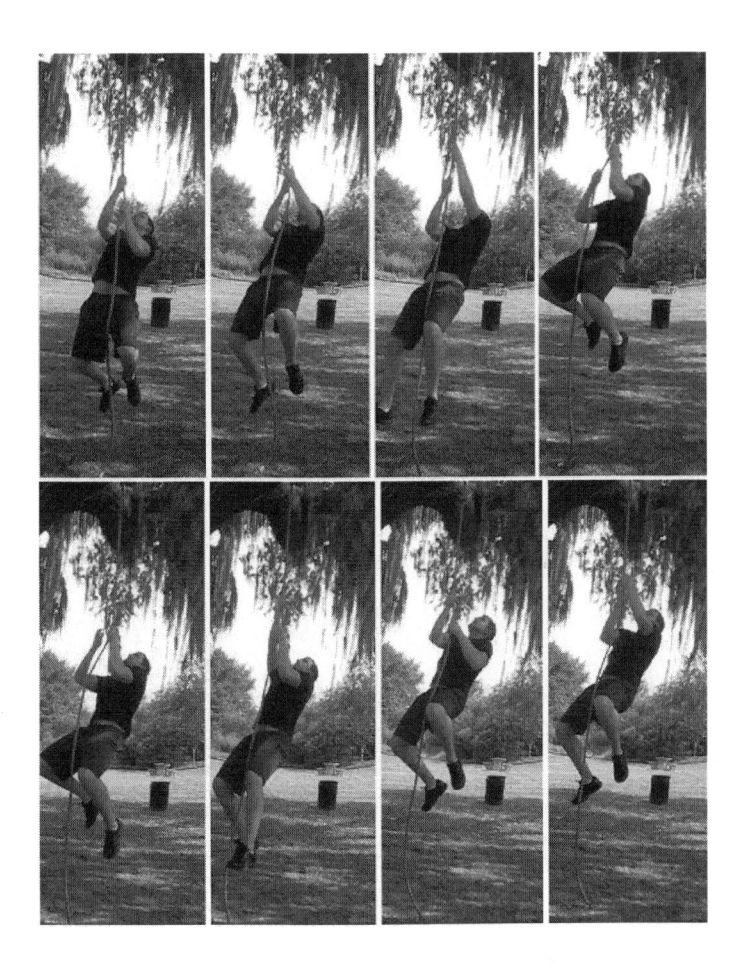

To lower yourself, simply reverse this process—and make sure you've got enough strength left "in the tank" to climb down in a safe, controlled manner.

When you first try this, don't go up more than one or two 'reaches.' Make sure you're comfortable getting down from that height before you try going any higher, so you know what you're getting into.

Rope climbing can be very rewarding, and it can help you to develop a pair of tough, strong hands that will help you in almost any strength activity.

You don't even need to be able to climb too high—as long as you can climb high enough to reach up at least once with each hand, you can climb repeatedly up and down with great results. Just take all reasonable precautions, don't get into any situation you aren't prepared for, and be sure to work both sides evenly.

ROLLING TOWELS

Did you ever think you could get one of the best hand and finger workouts ever... from a towel?

Neither did I, until I learned this exercise. This might be my favorite hand-strength specific exercise—because it's so unexpectedly effective—and if you keep at it, it will leave you with hands and forearms so sore you'll have trouble making a fist.

It's simple, but the details matter to make sure the exercise is as challenging as it should be. Let's start by looking at some pictures.

Start by finding any full-size towel. The longer, thicker, and heavier it is, the more difficult it will be, as you might imagine.

Then, hold the towel with both hands, straight out in front of you. Hold it from the top or bottom, with your arms

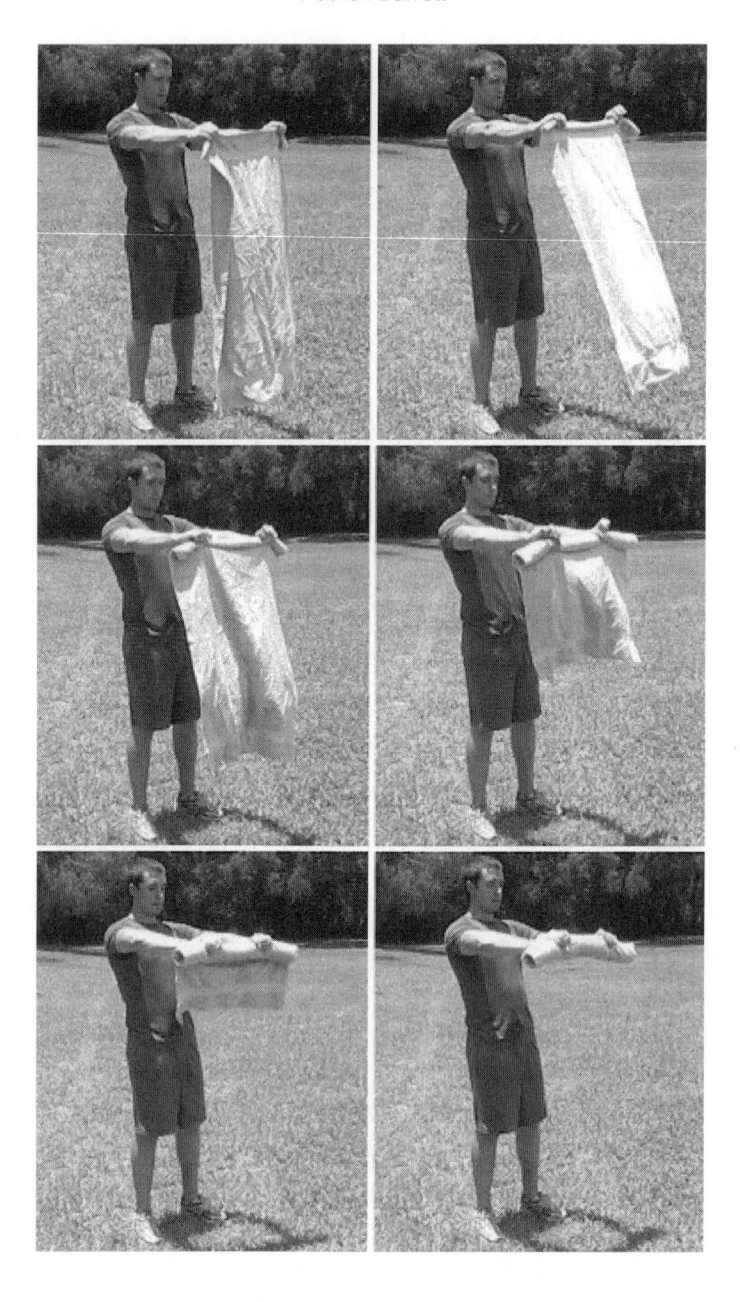

shoulder-width apart, between the thumb and forefinger of each hand.

Once you are in this position, start with both hands—simultaneously—to roll the towel up, all the way.

After you've rolled it up all the way, keep your arms straight out in front of you, and do the reverse, unrolling the towel back to the position you started in.

Finally, roll the towel up in the opposite direction (if you first rolled it forward/away from you, now roll it backward/toward you, or vice versa), and then again unroll back into the starting position. Repeat as much as you can.

This is a very challenging exercise, if you do it right. It requires you to use each finger individually, and since the rolled towel gets larger and smaller depending on where you are in the movement, it works out a full range of gripping positions, all without using any significant weight.

However, it is imperative that you follow good form to make sure that the exercise is properly challenging. In addition to what we've already talked about, you must make sure that both hands move at the same time. Don't roll one hand down, then hold it still while you roll with the other hand. Roll simultaneously in the same way; imagine that one hand is mirroring the other.

Also, try to keep all the movement in your wrists and hands. Your shoulders and elbows are bound to move a tiny bit, but minimize it as much as possible, and try to keep your arms as straight as possible.

Finally, don't neglect the unrolling part of the motion. It might be tempting to stop once the towel is rolled up and ignore the other half of the movement, especially because the unrolling is a little bit easier, but you'll get a better workout, both in your hands and in your shoulders, if you stay disciplined and stick to doing the entire exercise.

Once you get the form down, do the exercise—rolling it up, then unrolling it, then rolling it up the other way, then unrolling it, and so on—until you can't do it properly anymore. At first, that might happen pretty quickly, but soon you'll be able to go a few rounds before your shoulders can no longer keep your arms straight in front of you, and your fingers can no longer hold on to the towel.

If your hands are on the small side and you find you can't hold the towel toward the end as it gets larger, you have a few options. You may want to find a towel which is shorter, or (the better option) one that is thinner. You can also just roll it up as far as you're able to, then unroll from there, and so on.

For an extra challenge, try wetting the end of the towel—just an inch or so will be challenging, and obviously as you get stronger, you can wet it even more.

This is a truly outstanding forearm and hand strength exercise. Be sure to give it a shot, and take the time to get the form right. I learned this exercise studying the training materials of John Brookfield, one of the strongest grip-strength specialists ever (who I believe I mentioned earlier), so if you like it, you'll definitely enjoy his books, DVDs, and other materials.

SCHEDULE AND RECOVERY

Now that we've discussed all the different exercises, we need to talk about how you're going to incorporate them into your routine. Let me start out by saying that there are about 20 different exercises (including variations) in this book, and you should be sure to give every one of them a try if you're able to (obviously you can't climb a rope if you don't have a rope to climb, for example). Some of the these might be more effective than you think, so give each one a good chance.

Once you've tried out every exercise, you'll be in a better position to decide how to proceed. There are a lot of different ways to approach hand and forearm training. It can be as simple as picking 1-3 exercises from this book that you like, and adding them on to your normal upper body routine—typically 3-4 workouts a week with about a day of rest in between. That can be an effective and simple way to build stronger hands. You should rotate different exercises in and out, and always be sure to increase the difficulty as you get stronger so you keep making progress.

Another approach is to take some time (could be anywhere from 15 minutes to an hour or more) a few times a week to focus on making your hands and forearms stronger. Pick about 3-5 exercises to focus on, and move from one to the other. Most of these you do for as much time or as many repetitions as you can, so pick an exercise, do it until you can't anymore, take a minute to recover, then repeat that exercise. Do anywhere from one to five sets of that exercise in this way, then move to the next exercise, and continue like that.

You should stop your workout if you ever encounter any pain, but otherwise you can keep going until you can no longer perform the exercises with good form.

Still another approach, which can be used on its own or in conjunction with the two other approaches we just discussed, is just to fit in these workouts during the day. Many of these exercises can be done almost anywhere, especially if you're on a bus or a subway, or watching TV, or doing any other activity that doesn't require your hands and attention.

You can do your isometrics literally anywhere with no equipment at all—that by itself can really make your hands stronger. Or, you can use your gyro ball or grippers anywhere you bring them, and you can do broom walking and towel rolling when you're at home... the list goes on. So if you've got some time to kill and you want your hands to be stronger, don't be afraid to pick one of these exercises and do it.

Hand And Forearm Exercises

Anytime you do anything new, you'll find that you need more recovery time than usual, so if you're just getting started, feel free to wait until any soreness in your forearms is almost all gone before you do your next workout. However, as far as recovery in general is concerned, your hands and forearms are a little different from other parts of your body. They tend to recover from training more quickly.

A good rule of thumb is not to exercise your forearms too much if you have lingering soreness from your last workout (though a little soreness is okay). You might find, though, that you get good progress from having several days in a row of hand and forearm work—say, three or four days of hand exercises, followed by three or four days off, and so on.

As with most exercise, the most important thing is not the exact schedule you keep, just that you stick to some kind of schedule that makes you work hard—so find some version of what we've discussed in this chapter, add it to your routine, and make sure that you keep challenging yourself by increasing the difficulty and rotating in new exercises every so often.

And every few weeks, it's a good idea to take about a week off from any significant hand training, just to give your hands a good chance to recover, and to avoid injury.

CONNECT WITH ME

For further health, fitness, and nutrition information, you can find me online at BarrettBooks.com. You can read my blog posts and articles, including an ongoing series profiling strongmen, and another featuring common food additives.

You can also get in touch with me directly through the "Contact" page to ask me any exercise or nutrition question you might have, and I'll be happy to answer them as best I can in my "Training Q & A" section, where I answer questions from readers.

You'll see an e-mail sign-up form on the site as well where you can enter your e-mail address to stay up to date on blog posts and new books. You won't get e-mail more than about once a week, and of course I'll never spam you or sell your information, and you can unsubscribe at any time.

Another way to stay up to date is through my Facebook page, which can be found at Facebook.com/BarrettBooks.

I look forward to connecting with you, and please do contact me through my website with any questions or comments you might have.

CONCLUSION

Well, now you know everything you need to know to build exceptionally strong hands and forearms—all that's left is to go out there and do it.

This kind of training is easy to overlook, but it might be the one type of training whose benefits translate most directly into your ordinary daily life, whether that means playing organized sports, lifting weights, doing physical labor, or just getting around fulfilling ordinary responsbilities over the course of your day.

Your hands are one of your most important physical assets, so treat them right and make them strong. Use the isometrics. Make the block weights. Consider buying a gripper, or a gyro ball, or both.

And definitely, definitely, definitely do the towel rolling exercise. Trust me.

That about wraps things up. I hope you enjoyed this book, and I hope you learned some exercises that you'll put to use—why don't you put this book down and go try a few right now?

OTHER BOOKS BY PATRICK BARRETT

Natural Exercise*: Basic Bodyweight Training and Calisthenics for Strength and Weight-Loss*

Advanced Bodyweight Exercises*: An Intense Full Body Workout In A Home Or Gym*

The Natural Diet*: Simple Nutritional Advice For Optimal Health In The Modern World*

How To Do A Handstand*: From the Basic Exercises To The Free Standing Handstand Pushup*

Easy Exercises*: Simple Workout Routine For Busy People In The Office, At Home, Or On The Road*

Best Ab Exercises*: Abdominal Workout Routine For Core Strength And A Flat Stomach*

One Arm Pull Up*: Bodyweight Training And Exercise Program For One Arm Pull Ups And Chin Ups*

ABOUT THE AUTHOR

Patrick Barrett can be found on the web at BarrettBooks.com. He has been interested in exercise ever since he started to lift weights with his dad and older brothers as a kid. He participated in a half-dozen organized sports (most notably inline hockey and high school wrestling) until a neck injury during a wrestling match in his junior year prevented him from playing further in any contact sports.

After the injury, he developed an interest in pursuing strength and balance, particularly through bodyweight and self-taught gymnastic-type exercises.

Patrick has always loved both cooking and eating food. Unsatisfied with the confusing and often contradictory nutritional advice offered by mainstream sources, Patrick searched for another way to understand human nutrition that was logical, consistent, and effective. His books on food and nutrition reflect this 'cleaner,' more intuitive and useful understanding of food and how it impacts our health.

Patrick hopes that his books will save his audience time and aggravation by finally offering practical ways to achieve their nutrition and fitness goals.

Printed in Great Britain
by Amazon.co.uk, Ltd.,
Marston Gate.